Dissecting American Health Care

Commentaries on
Health, Policy, and Politics

Douglas B. Kamerow, MD

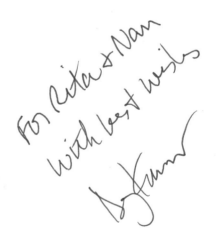

RTI Press

Library of Congress Control Number: 2011936221
ISBN 978-1-934831-06-9

RTI Press publication No. BK-0008-1109
doi:10.3768/rtipress.2011.bk.0008.1109
www.rti.org/rtipress.

The RTI Press mission is to disseminate information about RTI research, analytic tools, and technical expertise to a national and international audience. RTI Press publications are peer-reviewed by at least two independent substantive experts and one or more Press editors.

RTI International is an independent, nonprofit research organization dedicated to improving the human condition by turning knowledge into practice. RTI offers innovative research and technical services to governments and businesses worldwide in the areas of health and pharmaceuticals, education and training, surveys and statistics, advanced technology, international development, economic and social policy, energy and the environment, and laboratory testing and chemistry services.

This publication is part of the RTI Press Book series.
RTI International
3040 Cornwallis Road, PO Box 12194, Research Triangle Park, NC 27709-2194 USA
rtipress@rti.org
www.rti.org

Contents

Acknowledgments

Thanks to *BMJ* editors Richard Smith and Fiona Godlee for, respectively, hiring me and suggesting I do a regular column for the journal, and to my editor there, Trevor Jackson, for his continuing support and suggestions. Thanks to NPR's Ellen Silva for running my commentaries and teaching me how to write a piece "for the ear."

Thanks to my bosses at RTI, Al Miedema, Wayne Holden, and Jan Mitchell, for their support of this writing, both moral and financial. Thanks to the anonymous peer reviewers and to Kathleen Lohr and Karen Lauterbach at RTI Press for many helpful suggestions.

Thanks most to my wife, Celia Shapiro, the love of my life, and to our wonderful kids, Anna, Eli, and Simon. Best posse ever.

Introduction

I am a family doctor and preventive medicine specialist. I spent 20 years in the US Public Health Service working in a range of clinical, research, and policy positions, and then 10 years working at RTI International (formerly Research Triangle Institute) focusing on health services evaluations and health policy research. I also teach medical students and family medicine residents at Georgetown University.

Starting in 2007, I began to write short commentaries on health care and health policy for both the international medical journal *BMJ* (formerly the *British Medical Journal*) and the US radio and web network NPR (formerly National Public Radio—are we starting to see a trend to abbreviated names here?). Since then I have been producing an average of about 10 pieces a year. My goal in writing them has been to provide readers and listeners with thoughts and opinions on health-related issues, informed by evidence and experience. I also aimed to be interesting, provocative, and even entertaining.

The topics of the 47 essays included in this book are sometimes serious and sometimes lighthearted. They range from AIDS to screening tests for cancer to whether hair and nails grow after death. Not surprisingly, I have tended to write on subjects I know a bit about, hence an emphasis on primary care and preventive medicine. That has not stopped me from commenting on other areas, however, and so there are essays on ethics, genetics, and religion. In all cases I tried hard to get my facts straight before the pontifications began. (Speaking of pontifications, there is a piece about the pope as well.)

Because of the word limits necessary to fit onto a single medical journal page or into a typical 3-minute radio commentary, these are very short pieces. Whether this constraint has led to clear, concise writing that gets to the point quickly, or to superficial generalizations that only skim the surface of a topic, I leave to the reader's judgment.

The only thing these commentaries have in common is that they are all related to health or health care in some way. In retrospect, most were written in reaction to political events—an election or health reform—or policy pronouncements, such as a new screening test recommendation or an Institute of Medicine report. As I compiled them for this book I thought they fell fairly logically into five broad topic areas:

These last few years have been a boom time for evidence-based medicine, health care quality measurement, and quality improvement strategies. Essays in Section 1 focus on what works and what does not work in health care and how we can tell them apart.

Almost everyone thinks (wrongly) that virtually any kind of preventive medicine will save both lives and money. As a result, the early 21st century has been full of news and noise about clinical preventive services: screening tests, immunizations, and behavioral counseling. This is an area that I am dangerously knowledgeable about, and the second group of essays alternately praises and debunks trends in preventive care.

The US presidential campaign and election of 2008 fell right in the middle of this period. It provided delightful candidates and infuriating issues (or was it infuriating candidates and delightful issues?) to discuss and dissect. Section 3 focuses on politics and its intersection with health and health care. In it are profiles of interesting characters and discussions of soapbox issues like saving both primary care medicine and the surgeon general's purity.

When we look back on this period at mid-century, US health reform will no doubt be held up as a signal accomplishment—or failure. The US nonsystem of health care, with its perverse incentives and outrageous spending, has increasingly dominated the news in recent years. Section 4 is about the ups and downs of trying to change the way we deliver and pay for health care.

Although each of these short essays is an opinion piece, I have tried to keep myself out of the center of most of them. Sometimes, however, a personal experience became the backbone of the essay or seemed to introduce a subject well. These more personal pieces are grouped together with a few that deal with ethical issues in Section 5 at the end of the book. Forewarned is forearmed.

Within sections, the commentaries are sequenced chronologically, and the date originally published or broadcast is included at the top of each. This allows the reader to put date references such as "in January" or "on June 1" into context. It also reveals occasions when my crystal ball has been particularly cloudy, as when I gloomily predicted on January 30, 2010, that health care reform was doomed, less than 2 months before it passed and was signed into law. I have left these failed predictions as they were originally written.

All the essays are also labeled with their original source—NPR or *BMJ*. Because those written for the *BMJ* were styled for a medical journal, I have occasionally added footnotes to them to clarify medical or epidemiologic terms that might not be obvious to the general reader. Many of the sources I used in preparing these essays and all of the works I mention in the pieces themselves can be found in a bibliography at the end of the book.

1

Assessing and Improving Health Care

"Formerly, when religion was strong and science weak, men mistook magic for medicine; now, when science is strong and religion weak, men mistake medicine for magic."
—Thomas Szasz, MD, late 20th century psychiatrist and academic

When we look back on the last decade of the 20th century and the first decade of the 21st, they will likely be seen as a time in which we began to focus on improving the quality and safety of health care. Evidence-based medicine, another trend of this time, is part of the emphasis on quality improvement, but so is a careful look at processes of care. This first section of the book includes commentaries on how we can assess and improve health care.

Closely examining the nuts and bolts of how care is delivered is the first step to improving it. The first essay in this section discusses how a hospital has deconstructed a common procedure—cardiac bypass surgery—into its component parts to try to rationalize and improve it. They did this as part of an effort to "guarantee" a good outcome from the surgery for one preset price, quite a revolutionary approach. A subsequent commentary highlights an expansion of the typically hospital-based quality improvement movement into the outpatient setting. Medical errors are no less prevalent in the office than they are in the hospital, but they are harder to document. Only by discovering and categorizing these mistakes of omission and commission can we begin to prevent them.

Three commentaries in this section discuss recent trends in American health care. Retail health clinics, located in the back of drug stores and "big box" establishments like Wal-Mart, are offering convenient locations and hours and little or no waiting time to see nurse practitioners for acute medical problems. Will they serve as a useful adjunct to primary care or are they a threat to replace it? Similarly, alternative medicine providers and therapies are increasing rapidly in almost every part of the country, offering very popular but largely unproven therapies and preventatives to patients who mainly pay cash for them. Third, a trend toward nonsurgical hospital-only specialists, called hospitalists, is also spreading rapidly. Hospitals are trying to maximize efficiency and profits while many primary care doctors are glad to be relieved of the need to make hospital rounds every day. All three of these trends raise questions about quality and continuity of care.

New medical technologies are either going to save us or bankrupt us—or maybe both. One problem is how to determine whether promising technologies are beneficial when some people are already using them. The Centers for Medicare & Medicaid Services in the US has come up with a process—called "coverage with evidence development"—that allows for special Medicare coverage of some of these new procedures while enrolling the patient in a clinical trial or register to keep track of whether it works or not. This both improves our knowledge of what works and potentially helps some patients right away.

The biggest success or disappointment in the last decade—again, depending on how you see it—has got to be genetic medicine. Since we completed the decoding of the human genome in 2003, geneticists have been promising major improvements in how we diagnose and treat diseases. Generally this is spoken about in terms of personalized medicine, where we each get treatments that match our genetic make-up and thus are immediately suitable for our constitutions.

So far, medicine generally has not delivered on this genetic promise. The good news, however, is that Congress did finally pass legislation outlawing discrimination based on genetic risk for specific diseases, which was one of the concerns in my commentary on the subject.

Also included in this section are two more lighthearted pieces, based on articles by two Indiana University doctors who expose medical myths that our mothers (and sometimes our doctors) have told us. It is good to review these to find out what not to pass on to our own children.

BMJ, May 26, 2007

Great health care, guaranteed

A 90-day guarantee on surgery may be the first step to improving quality

A recent front page story in the *New York Times* described a health care system in Pennsylvania that has been giving a 90-day guarantee on its coronary artery bypass surgeries since February 2006. For a fixed price, patients get the operation, postoperative care, and any necessary follow-up treatment, including rehospitalization and even repeat surgery. There are no extra charges. This is news in America, where we are used to unit pricing in health care. That generally leads, of course, to a perverse incentive: if you do a poor job and extra care is needed, you get paid more.

The newspaper likened the surgical guarantee to a warranty on a new car or a home appliance. The health care system, Geisinger, guarantees that all will go well or it will fix the problem, at no additional cost to the purchaser … er … patient. I generally don't like using the term "consumer" for patients, but in this case it seems appropriate. The customer is buying a product, coronary artery grafts, and the installer of the product, the hospital, stands behind its work. Sort of like a brake job at the auto repair shop, but a little more complicated and a lot less mechanical.

Bypass graft surgery is generally a big winner financially for American hospitals; they make money on them and try to increase their volume to make more money. So, for the guarantee plan to pay off in our medical economy, Geisinger has to price the surgery competitively and keep costs in line. To do that, it has to minimize expensive adverse outcomes. And to deliver good surgical outcomes on a regular basis, the health system has to do two things: identify the "right" processes—those that are linked to good outcomes—and deliver them consistently.

To identify the right things to do, Geisinger staff reviewed the American College of Cardiology/American Heart Association guidelines and operationalized them into 40 best practices and benchmarks. These cover everything from preadmission screening to post-discharge care. They then incorporated the best practices into all hospital processes and procedures.

Prompts and defaults were programmed into electronic health records, for example, and surgery was automatically cancelled if specific benchmarks weren't met.

It took a while to get everyone on board. Herding surgeons is probably as difficult as herding cats. Even after all parties agreed to the benchmarks, only 60 percent were actually being met. After three months, the percentage reached 100 percent, and it remained above 90 percent throughout the first year.

How has it worked? Reasonably well. A year into the project, Geisinger staff presented a comparison of their 2005 and 2006 elective bypass surgery outcomes at a surgical society meeting. The trends are all going in the right direction: more patients with no complications, fewer blood transfusions, decreased operative mortality, and fewer pulmonary complications. Most improvements are not yet statistically significant, owing to small numbers, but the results are promising. Length of stay has decreased by 12 percent and hospital charges have fallen by 5 percent. The elusive goal of decreasing costs while increasing quality seems to be within reach for this procedure.

The Geisinger story shows that it takes a huge amount of work to optimize all the aspects of care for even one type of surgery, much less for all operations or for everything that happens in a hospital or an outpatient clinic. A lot of the quality improvement work that has gone on so far in the US has been less ambitious. It is usually what might be called the "quality nugget" approach— find one isolated thing that has been shown to make a difference, figure out some way to do it or not do it, measure the results, and declare victory. So we have lists and lists of "quality measures" that tend to round up the usual suspects: beta blocker drugs and statins after heart attacks, support stockings or low-molecular-weight heparin when the patient is immobilized, eye and foot examinations for people with diabetes, and so forth.

It is worth looking back at the impetus for the medical errors/quality crusade in the US: the Institute of Medicine reports of 1999 (*To Err Is Human*) and 2001 (*Crossing the Quality Chasm*). The first report documented the shocking costs, in morbidity and mortality, of medical errors; showed how other industries had dealt with similar problems; and recommended a systematic approach to document and analyze errors and improve patient safety. The latter expanded the focus from patient safety to health care quality. It proposed a comprehensive re-imagining of how evidence-based health care is delivered: customized to patients' needs in a transparent health care system where safety is a system property, waste is continuously decreased, knowledge is shared, and outcomes are optimized.

We are obviously not there yet. But to get there we need to move beyond the piecemeal quality nugget approach to a much more comprehensive redesign of the systems that deliver health care and of the training received by the people who work in them. As quality guru Don Berwick said in the *New York Times* article, "Getting everything right is really, really hard." It seems to me that the Geisinger bypass surgery program is both an admirable first step and a scary example of how difficult it will be to totally reinvent medical care.

BMJ, July 7, 2007

Retail health clinics—threat or promise?

In the US, a health clinic increasingly may be in the back of a store

American doctors are up in arms about retail-based clinics. Hundreds have opened, located in about half the states. Last week, the American Medical Association House of Delegates beat back a proposal by some worried members to call for a ban on the clinics. They did, however, adopt a resolution asking state and federal authorities to investigate whether these low price, convenient competitors were putting patients at risk.

Most retail clinics are located near the prescription counter inside large grocery stores or pharmacies. They are open long hours 7 days a week. They are staffed by nurse practitioners or physician assistants who diagnose and treat common illnesses, give immunizations, do physical examinations, and perform a limited number of procedures.

Unlike in the UK, where some GPs have set up walk-in centers in retail settings, the US clinics are usually not full-service clinics staffed by doctors. Nor are they owned by doctors or hospitals. Most are owned by one of a dozen for-profit companies, with up to 200 clinics each.

As Richard Bohmer pointed out earlier this year, the organizing principles of these clinics are taken right from the fast food industry: convenient locations, long opening hours, limited menu, low prices, and consistent (if not always the highest) quality. As opposed to sorting by urgency (as an emergency department does) or by body part or system (as doctors do), retail clinics stratify by complexity. Anything that can be done by mid-level practitioners based on well accepted guidelines is in. Anything that involves too much judgment, ongoing chronic care, or serious consequences is referred out.

Patients love them. A recent national poll found that between 80 percent and 90 percent of users were satisfied with the quality of care, convenience, and costs of the centers. The leading factors behind patients' selection of a retail health center over an emergency room or doctor's office in an Arizona poll were (in order) convenient location, walk-in (no appointment) policy, and short waiting time.

One Sunday afternoon, I visited my local Minute Clinic to check it out. I drove 5 minutes to a large pharmacy in Bethesda, Maryland, parked in the free lot, walked in, and headed to the back of the store. I found the small waiting area empty, with a sign saying that the nurse practitioner was in one of the two examination rooms with a patient. I signed in and sat down.

While I waited, a large flat-screen video display flashed promotional material alternating with the menu of services: common illnesses (ear and eye infections, bladder infections, allergies) $49 to $59; skin conditions (minor sunburn, poison ivy, athlete's foot) $49; vaccines $30 to $110. The clinic takes cash and credit cards, and accepts most health insurance plans. Thus, you pay either the listed price or (if your insurance is accepted) a smaller co-payment.

After about 5 minutes, a pleasant, middle-aged nurse practitioner came out and greeted me. I asked her to check if my insurance was honored. It wasn't. I told her I'd think about it, and she turned to the customer (patient?) who had signed in after me, greeted him, and took him into an examination room to determine the appropriateness of his complaint. I tried to overhear what was going on but couldn't. I picked up some literature and left.

These clinics clearly work for people who have an acute, limited problem or need an immunization or other offered service, as long as they also have the means or insurance to pay for it. Perfect for a child's recurrent ear infection on a Sunday or an assessment of painful urination in the evening. Quick examination, diagnosis, treatment, and the prescription can be filled without moving your car. Or if you're on vacation and develop conjunctivitis or a sinus infection, nothing could be more convenient.

But legitimate clinical questions exist. Where is the medical back-up? What do they do when a true emergency walks in? How do you sort out the simple, minor problem from the serious problem presenting with common symptoms? The clinics answer that they hire certified, experienced nurse practitioners who know what they are doing and when to get help. They follow recognized guidelines in the diagnosis and treatment of the disorders they treat. They triage each patient to make sure that the problem is within scope; if it's not, they refer them to their own doctor or another doctor, with no charge for the visit. All the clinics have telephone backup with a doctor, although sometimes that doctor is in another state. As for emergencies, they really don't see many. Most patients understand what these clinics can do and can't do and triage themselves accordingly.

Economic questions also exist, of course. Are these clinics providing quick, competent, convenient care, relieving busy doctors from having to deal with mild acute illnesses so they can focus on more complex and important problems? Or are they "cream skimming," taking all the lucrative brief visits by insured patients and leaving the miserable poor to fill up doctors' waiting rooms? The answer depends on who you ask.

Certainly the retail health clinics are a threat. But they are providing a useful service, from which conventional practitioners could learn a thing or two. In that sense they provide additional impetus for medicine to reinvent itself to become more patient-centered and responsive.

BMJ, September 29, 2007

CAM to the rescue

Alternative medicine is wildly popular, but what are we supposed to do about it?

I got a phone call the other day from a man asking whether I did "alternative" medicine. When I told him that I wasn't in regular practice, he asked for a referral to someone who could provide this type of care. It made me think.

Complementary and alternative medicine (CAM) comprises a diverse group of treatments, ranging from symptomatic interventions to be used in conjunction with traditional therapies—therapeutic touch or meditation—to unique treatments meant to replace conventional chemotherapy or surgery. CAM includes complex and longstanding systems of care, such as acupuncture, ayurvedic medicine, and homeopathy, but it can also be as straightforward as taking a specific dietary supplement to lower blood pressure or blood lipid concentrations.

Americans love CAM. Over a third of us report having used some form of CAM therapy in the previous 12 months, and use is increasing every year. Leading CAM therapies include natural products (supplements and herbal medicines), meditation, chiropractic, and massage. Symptoms most commonly treated with CAM therapies include musculoskeletal, respiratory, and psychological symptoms.

It's a huge business. Americans spend at least $50 billion a year on CAM therapies. An increasing amount of this care is covered by health insurance, although generally this applies only to the more accepted CAM treatments, such as acupuncture and chiropractic. About a third to a half of all spending on CAM is paid out of patients' pockets, more than we pay directly for hospitalizations.

Despite all this, many Americans don't like to talk to their conventional doctors about the CAM treatments they are using. Only about a third to a half of patients who use CAM report discussing this with their doctor. Their reasons vary from thinking that doctors will not be supportive to saying that it is not important for doctors to know. That's a potential problem, given the documented interactions between some natural products and conventional drugs. Surveys in the US find that doctors rarely ask about use of CAM products, even though they admit they need to know more about them.

With all of this activity, it would be nice to know which CAM treatments work and which do not. A number of Cochrane reviews have looked at CAM treatments, and the US Agency for Healthcare Research and Quality has commissioned around 20 evidence reports—systematic reviews—on CAM therapies. The UK's National Institute for Health and Clinical Excellence (NICE) has explicitly avoided assessing CAM, however, despite calls for it to do so.

In response to a mandate from Congress, the National Institutes of Health created the National Center for Complementary and Alternative Medicine in 1999. Its mission is to support rigorous research into CAM and to disseminate its results. This research ranges from large randomized controlled trials of CAM products to basic science research to elucidate physiological explanations for CAM therapies such as acupuncture and ayurvedic medicine. The center has spent hundreds of millions of dollars investigating CAM products and treatments.

So why don't we know more than we do about what works and what doesn't? Part of the explanation is the huge number and heterogeneity of CAM interventions. Only a small number of the most promising treatments have so far been rigorously tested. Part of the problem is the nature of CAM treatments: they can be hard to quantify and hard to specify, and often they don't lend themselves to standard research techniques such as placebo-controlled trials.

Furthermore, once research is done, it is often hard to assess its quality. Paul Shekelle and colleagues have written about the difficulties of systematically reviewing CAM studies. The challenges include various biases that CAM studies are prone to; difficulty in locating the literature; treatment variability; variability in use of comparison placebo or sham treatments; and dealing with rare but serious adverse events.

Critics say that CAM doesn't deserve a place at the table—that enough time has passed and enough research has been done to show whether any of these interventions are safe and effective. The fact that unequivocal success stories exist indicates only that the treatments are placebo and expectation effects masquerading as medicine, they insist. And yet so many people use them and seem to derive benefit, it seems a shame to lump them all together and throw them out.

I think a sensible approach is, first, for doctors to inquire of patients what nontraditional treatments they are using, both for conditions that the doctor knows about and is treating and for others that have not been addressed. This would at least allow discussion and investigation of possible adverse interactions. Second, doctors should discuss truly complementary symptomatic CAM treatments—for chronic pain, allergies, or the like—so that their scientific basis can be investigated and understood by the patient and the doctor, if possible. Third, for alternative treatments prescribed for serious or life threatening diseases such as cancer, doctors should assess the scientific evidence for the treatment and try to understand the range of benefit the patient expects to receive from it.

We all need to pay more attention to the CAM treatments that patients are seeking out and are willing to pay for, and to the evidence behind their effectiveness.

BMJ, November 10, 2007

Paying for promising but unproven technologies

Is the policy on "coverage with evidence development" a helpful way forward?

Promising new medical technologies, especially expensive ones, pose a difficult problem for health care systems. If there is not enough evidence for conventional systematic reviews and technology assessments to find benefit, the default decision is that a new technology, whether drug, device, or surgical procedure, is not "covered" and thus not paid for. This seems reasonable when we are talking about a screening test or other preventive maneuver, since most would agree that we should require a high level of proof before exposing a well population to expensive and potentially harmful interventions. But what about when the person is sick, perhaps with advanced cancer, and the promising technology is a potentially lifesaving chemotherapeutic agent, a new surgical procedure, or a drug already approved but for a different condition?

On the other hand, to allow payment for all such technologies might break the bank if the new interventions are expensive, and of course they may not work at all. Everyone's favorite cautionary example is high-dose chemotherapy with autologous bone marrow transplantation for advanced breast cancer. Hugely expensive but thought to be helpful, it was the subject of intense scrutiny and publicity in the US about 10 years ago. Many women with advanced breast cancer demanded that their health insurance plans cover the procedure and sued the companies in court when they did not. Only when a definitive randomized controlled trial found no benefit did the furor subside.

It seems that a middle ground between "yes" and "no" is needed in situations in which new technologies have suggestive but not definitive evidence of benefit, especially when they are thought to be breakthroughs or highly cost-effective treatments. Such a coverage option was first developed in the US in 1995 in response to another then-promising technology, lung volume reduction surgery (LVRS) for chronic obstructive lung disease. US government staff in the Medicare program, which pays for care for elderly people and some disabled patients, noticed a dramatic increase in insurance payments for this expensive and dangerous surgery in the early and mid-1990s. Surgical centers had developed a new, safer technique for the operation and were claiming great success in patients with end-stage lung disease, allowing them to walk about and live much more normal lives again after surgery. A government-sponsored technology assessment, however, could find no supportive randomized evidence for the procedure, leading to a national noncoverage decision. This unleashed a political firestorm.

In 1995, Medicare announced an innovative response to this situation: it would cover LVRS, but only if patients consented to be randomized into a multicenter trial sponsored by the National Institutes for Health comparing the surgery with optimal medical treatment. Medicare called this policy "coverage with evidence development." The LVRS study was a challenging trial to perform, with much public controversy played out in the news media and even in Congress, but ultimately some 1,200 patients were randomized. When the results were published, LVRS showed no overall survival advantage to intensive medical treatment, but selective improvements were seen in exercise capacity and quality of life for certain patients. The trial also highlighted the true risks of the surgery, as perioperative mortality was almost 10 percent. Although Medicare ultimately covered LVRS in selected patients, the trial results scared most referring doctors and patients away from it, and it has been largely abandoned in the past 5 years.

Is it ethical to demand that patients who want a procedure be forced to enroll in a trial in which they are equally as likely to receive a control intervention as the treatment they are seeking? Lawyers, often representing the technology developers or "denied" patients, have argued that coverage with evidence development policies are coercive, unfair, and illegal. Ethicists disagree, as long as the technologies are chosen carefully and appropriately and the policies provide a net increase in coverage for technologies that would otherwise be denied approval.

Medicare staff have subsequently refined and reissued their policy on coverage with evidence development and more carefully justified its legal basis. It has been used to provide limited coverage for carotid artery angioplasty with stenting and for PET (positron emission tomography) scanning in the evaluation of dementia patients, both in the context of clinical trials. Most recently, the policy was used to mandate that expanded coverage of implantable cardioverter-defibrillators for prevention of sudden death be linked with patient enrollment in an ongoing national data register, which will allow assessment of who benefits from this technology and who does not.

The US experience with this issue was not lost on the UK Department of Health when it set up the National Institute for Health and Clinical Excellence (NICE) in 1999. It provided for a NICE recommendation category termed "approval only in the context of research" or OIR, which has been used sparingly since NICE was initiated. Kalipso Chalkidou and colleagues have recently reviewed the NICE experience with OIR recommendations. They conclude that OIR, when used sparingly, has provided an important alternative to a "yes" or "no" decision on the appropriateness of technologies. But they concede that they face twin challenges similar to their US (and indeed, worldwide) colleagues: developing a clear and reproducible set of criteria for when to use coverage with evidence development, and ensuring the timeliness and funding of the research studies they recommend.

BMJ, January 5, 2008

Waiting for the genetic revolution

Will 2008 be the year that genomics delivers on its promises?

The sequencing of the human genome was completed in 2003. Since then we've been told that we're living in the "genomic era"—the biggest revolution in human health since antibiotics, some say, and the beginning of scientific, personalized medicine.

In the United States we've spent about $4 billion since 2000 to fund the National Human Genome Research Institute, so it seems fair to ask what we've gotten for our money.

Certainly there have been dramatic improvements in the efficiency of DNA sequencing and other related technologies. Polymerase chain reaction and other amplification techniques have made what was exotic and painstaking work commonplace and quick. And I guess that some indirect applications of genomics can be found in the doctor's office. Human papillomavirus DNA testing, rapid tests for some infectious diseases by polymerase chain reaction, HIV analyses, and other diagnostic laboratory tests have found their way into general practice.

Genomic tools have been used to develop some drugs that specialists use, and more are being evaluated all the time. But most that I've heard of are the province of oncologists or ophthalmologists. Given that we baby boomers are all getting older, I suppose I should be happy that new drugs are available for age-related macular degeneration, arthritis, and various cancers, but I'm not sure how big a difference they've made on a population basis.

Pharmacogenomic testing may be able to help us target specific drugs at the people most likely to benefit from them, telling us who should get trastuzumab (if they can afford it), who is likely to be hypersensitive to which antiretroviral, or which chemotherapy regimen is likely to be most effective. But again this is specialist-level stuff.

What about the common, everyday diagnoses—heart disease, diabetes, and other multi-gene disorders? I hope that there is some new information out about them. Generally when I hear experts addressing primary care doctors on genomics they offer the same stock examples: the woman with breast and cervical cancer in her family history who is referred with her daughters for testing; the man with colorectal cancer at a young age who turns out to have a hereditary syndrome. But we knew about these kinds of things a long time ago—we just didn't have the exact gene. It comes down to taking a good family history.

Maybe the future lies in the flashy new genetic testing websites that have sprung up, all planning to start collecting our money and DNA this year. Just pay your $995 to $2500, spit into a tube or scrape your cheek, and in four to six weeks you can see your genetic destiny on a special secure website. Apparently the smart money is betting on these companies, to judge from the venture capitalists they have behind them, including Google founder Sergey Brin and Silicon Valley guru Esther Dyson.

These "personal genomic services" allow you to "unlock the secrets of your own DNA." They can tell you your risk of developing lots of common and less common diseases, in comparison with the rest of the population. The rub, of course, is what to do with these data. All the sites take pains to point out that they aren't giving medical advice. And most of them don't report any single-gene disorders that are the daily work of clinical geneticists and genetic counselors. What are you supposed to do with the knowledge that you have a 30 percent increased risk of Alzheimer's disease or a 40 percent decreased likelihood of developing atrial fibrillation? Change your behavior? How?

There is precious little evidence that simple knowledge about anything changes people's health-related behaviors. And even less is known about how people's knowledge of their genetic risks will affect them. The Centers for Disease Control and Prevention convened a panel of experts in 2004 to assess genetic tests and technologies for their appropriateness in practice. After 3 years of work setting up a systematic, evidence-based process, they have just issued their first recommendation. They evaluated pharmacogenomic testing for cytochrome P450 in depressed patients to predict how well selective serotonin reuptake inhibitors would work. Their conclusion: the evidence to recommend for or against such testing is insufficient.

And what about all the legal and ethical challenges involved in genetic testing, especially the broad genetic surveys? It's probably not an accident that these new websites steer clear of conventional medical care. What will happen if (or when) insurance companies get hold of our genetic profiles? Legislation that would prohibit discrimination on the basis of genetic risks has been pending at the US Congress for a number of years but never seems to pass. It is no surprise that the US National Human Genome Research Institute has a whole program devoted to research and policies on what they call "ELSI," the ethical, legal, and social issues involved in genomics.

This is not to say that progress hasn't been made or that these discoveries won't someday revolutionize health care. But the day when the genome is a regular part of the medical record, when personalized medicine is a reality rather than a catchphrase, still seems a long way off.

NPR, January 10, 2008

Separating medical truth from fiction

Don't believe everything your doctor tells you

One of the things I like best about the British medical journal *BMJ* is its humor and irreverent style. A great example of this is a recent article by two Indiana University doctors, Rachel Vreeman and Aaron Carroll. They critically examined some strongly held medical beliefs that you may have heard from your mother or even from your doctor. They're not quite true.

For example, take "reading in dim light ruins your eyesight." If you spent your childhood reading with a flashlight under the covers, you can rest assured. Although poor lighting can cause glinting and dry eyes temporarily, there's no evidence that any permanent damage is done. When you think about it, lighting has only improved since the days when everyone read by candlelight, and vision hasn't gotten any better. In fact, near-sightedness is more common these days with better lighting.

Or how about the old saw that we only use 10 percent of our brains? This one, apparently, has been around since the turn of the last century, and it's been attributed to Albert Einstein. Modern medical imaging, however, shows that we use much more than 10 percent of our brains. Essentially no areas of the brain are completely inactive, and studies of people with brain injuries have found that damage to virtually any part of the brain is associated with specific and lasting negative effects.

Okay, here's one that everyone knows is true: shaving causes hair to grow back faster or coarser. If you're a woman, I guarantee someone has told you this at least once. For this one, we have strong evidence that it's a myth. Clinical trials have proven that shaving has no effect on the rate of hair growth or on the thickness of the hair that grows back. What unshaven hair does have is a finer taper at the end, which may make it look less coarse. And newly grown hair looks darker because the sun hasn't had a chance to bleach it.

Speaking of hair, have you ever been told that hair and fingernails continue to grow even after someone dies? What's going on here, it turns out, is that post-mortem drying of the skin can cause it to retract around the hair and nails, making it look like they're growing. But there's no way that the hair and nails actually continue to grow without the ongoing delivery of nutrients that a beating heart delivers.

Finally, how many diet articles and books have you read that advocate drinking at least eight glasses of water a day? No one knows exactly where this one came from, but it might be from a leading nutritionist in 1970s. It turns out that there is no such requirement. Thirst is the best guide for how much you need to drink. Further, drinking liquids in excessive amounts can actually be dangerous, as we see in the occasional marathon runner who over-drinks, gets water intoxication, and dies.

Bottom line? Don't believe everything your mother, or maybe even your doctor, tells you.

NPR, August 20, 2008

Testing errors in the doctor's office

Medical errors don't just happen in the hospital

When we think about medical errors and patient safety, we generally envision hospital disasters like cutting off the wrong leg in surgery or giving the wrong medicine in an IV that stops someone's heart. That's because, first, these are dramatic and unacceptable events, and second because almost all the research on patient safety so far has been done in inpatient hospital settings.

This is changing. A network of family doctors, sponsored by the American Academy of Family Physicians and the federal Agency for Healthcare Research and Quality, is bravely reporting on and analyzing medical errors in doctors' offices. One of their recent studies focused on medical tests.

Medical tests include blood tests and imaging studies like X-rays, as well as Pap smears and other, more procedural tests. Errors can occur throughout the testing process: the wrong test can be ordered, the wrong test can be done, or the results can get lost or misfiled. The doctor can misinterpret the test, not notify the patient of the results, or give the wrong advice. This study looked at the whole continuum of testing and analyzed almost 1,000 errors in eight family medicine practices.

About a quarter of the errors were related to reporting test results to the doctor—they were incomplete, late, or lost. The next two leading causes were errors in test implementation—the wrong test was done or the specimen was lost—and administrative errors, usually related to mistakes in filing the results or putting them into the patient's medical record. All together, these three kinds of problems accounted for more than 60 percent of the errors.

Most of the consequences of the errors were inefficiency and inconvenience: lost time, greater costs, and delays in care, none of which affected the patient's health. But 18 percent of the errors led to physical or emotional harm, so there are important consequences to these mistakes. Doctors can use research like this to improve the systems in their practices, so that the testing process is less likely to fail. Patients should take away from these studies the importance of being involved in their care.

Bottom line? When your doctor orders tests for you, make a note of which tests they are so that you can check when you get them that the correct test is being performed. If you don't hear back from the doctor's office about the results, give them a call to follow up. Make sure that the right tests were done and that you know the results and what they mean for you and your health.

NPR, December 24, 2008

Scientists shed light on festive medical myths

Science trumps our traditions

Indiana University doctors Rachel Vreeman and Aaron Carroll have debunked a group of health-related myths in another article in the medical journal *BMJ*. As we approach the end of the year and its attendant celebrations, bear in mind these scientific findings.

First of all, if you have children or pets, you don't have to worry anymore about having poinsettias around your house. Despite long-standing beliefs to the contrary, poinsettia leaves and flowers are not poisonous. Toxicity studies in rats and reviews of poison control center data about human ingestion have failed to find any toxic level of poinsettia.

Here is one that will make your kids happy: eating sugar and sweets does not make children hyperactive. Although countless parents will disagree, at least a dozen carefully controlled studies have failed to find any effect of dietary sugar on children's behavior. Some of these studies were even done on so-called hyperactive kids, who were thought to be at greater risk for this reaction.

It turns out that at least part of the problem is parental expectations. This was confirmed by a study that had parents score their children's behavior after they consumed what the parents thought was a sugary drink. Even when the drink contained no sugar, the parents rated their kids' behavior as hyperactive. So, bring on the sugarplums.

On a more serious note, the common wisdom that suicides are more frequent during the winter holiday season is also false. Studies done around the world have failed to find a spike in suicide rates during the holidays or during the cold, dark winter months. Suicide levels peak at different times in different countries among people of different ages, but there is no consistent pattern.

Speaking of cold weather, how many times have you heard that you "lose most of your body heat through your head"? My mother certainly told me that, and even the US Army survival manual tells us that soldiers lose "40 to 45 percent" of body heat through their heads.

But recent studies have debunked this old soldier's tale. Any uncovered part of the body loses heat and will drop the core body temperature proportionately.

If you walk outside in winter with a hat on but wearing shorts, you're going to be cold.

Finally, for New Year's Eve, what's your favorite nostrum to prevent or treat a hangover? Bananas? Aspirin? Burnt toast? Raw eggs? Black coffee? Surprisingly few scientific studies have been done on hangover medicines and, unfortunately, no scientific evidence supports any cure for drinking too much. Some studies in rats show promising potential treatments, but nothing is ready for prime time yet.

Bottom line? Drink alcohol in moderation if you don't want a hangover. And have a happy, healthy new year.

NPR, March 12, 2009

Hospitalists—a new kind of doctor

The pros and cons of having a specialist hospital doctor

Suppose you get very sick and you need to be hospitalized. In the old days, your doctor would take care of you in the hospital, writing the orders for your medicines, making rounds every day, asking specialists to see you. But now the management of your hospital care may be transferred to a new type of specialist who takes care of hospitalized patients only. What's going on?

Researchers from the University of Texas analyzed 10 years of Medicare data and found that these hospital-only doctors, called hospitalists, are growing at a rate of almost 30 percent a year. In some parts of the country, they take care of 70 or even 80 percent of hospitalized Medicare patients. This is a huge change, and it has important implications.

Why is this happening? In a word: efficiency. Since hospitals generally get paid one fee for each hospitalization, they want to get patients home as soon as possible. They have found that it is more efficient to have doctors in the hospital all the time to make decisions and move things along, rather than waiting for your doctor to make rounds once a day. Also, since payments for primary care doctors have gone down, they need to see more and more patients in their offices in order to make a living. Going to the hospital every day cuts into that time and isn't very cost-effective for them if they only have a few hospitalized patients.

There are other reasons for hospital-only doctors besides efficiency, though. Hospitalists arguably should provide better care, not just faster care, since they are always available and spend all of their time focusing on inpatient problems. Research hasn't proven that patients who have hospital-only doctors do better, but there are some studies leaning that way. It is also logical to assume that doctors who spend all their time taking care of hospitalized patients will know more about hospital systems and quality improvement programs than primary care doctors do.

There are serious concerns about this hospital-only doctor movement as well, and they mainly revolve around "transitions." These occur when patients are admitted to the hospital and when they go home. The hospital doctor, no matter how smart or experienced, isn't going to know you or your history or your problems. It's crucially important that your doctor communicate extensively with the hospital doctor about all these things when you are admitted.

Similarly, when it is time to go home, especially if you are still somewhat sick and need close monitoring, your primary care doctor needs to know what happened, how you're doing, and what medicines you're on in order to resume caring for you. This is where things break down and the new system can have potentially catastrophic effects. Health reform and increased use of electronic medical records will help these transitions, but there still is no substitute for close communication.

Bottom line? If you are going to be admitted to the hospital, insist that your records go with you and that your doctor personally talks with the doctor or doctors who will be managing your care, before *and after* your hospitalization.

2

Preventive Medicine

"An ounce of prevention is worth a pound of cure."

—17th century proverb

"An ounce of prevention is a ton of work."

—Paul Frame, MD, late 20th century prevention expert

The essays in this section all discuss clinical preventive services: screening tests for the early detection of disease, immunizations, and counseling to change risky health-related behaviors. Included are pieces about the preventive services that are often in the headlines, like mammograms, prostate cancer screening, and flu shots. In addition, other commentaries address preventive care that usually does not get much attention but should: routine childhood immunizations, hypertension screening, and depression screening. The re-emergence of measles as a cause of illness and even death was something I wrote about in 2008, and it is in the headlines again as I write this introduction, 3 years later.

Sometimes preventive care recommendations are controversial, especially when they fly in the face of common sense. Just because a disease is common and deadly does not mean we should screen everyone for it. What we really want to know is whether the preventive maneuver actually makes a difference in the patient's clinical outcome for that condition. We are lucky to have good evidence about many of these services, as well as evidence-based guidelines on their use. The very first essay in the section discusses the vexing problem of whether there is enough evidence to recommend routine screening of children for elevated blood cholesterol levels, thus committing those found by screening to a lifetime of treatment. Personal preferences sometimes play an important role as well, especially when the evidence is inconclusive about whether the screening test does more good than harm.

As the evidence changes, so do evidence-based guidelines. An essay on lung cancer screening discusses new research that is likely to lead to changes in practice and, ultimately, in health outcomes from what is still the leading cause of cancer deaths. A commentary on the 30th anniversary of AIDS describes recent work proving that what was once good treatment has now become effective preventive care as well.

Costs also enter into the discussion of preventive medicine, as these services are often held up as cost-saving by well-meaning politicians and others. As an essay on this topic points out, though, the proper question to ask about preventive care—and any health care, for that matter—is not whether the specific service saves money. Rather, it is whether it provides good value in terms of health outcomes for the particular population in question.

BMJ, July 26, 2008

Should we screen for childhood dyslipidemia?

The obesity epidemic raises the stakes for using statins in children

It is not an accident that evidence-based guidelines more or less began with clinical preventive services. Unlike treatment for problems that produce symptoms, preventive medicine is optional. We have the luxury of time to gather and evaluate the evidence for the efficacy and even effectiveness* of screening tests and counseling. When someone rushes into a doctor's office bleeding or doubled over in pain, it would hardly be acceptable to send them away untreated to await the results of a randomized controlled trial for their problem. But that is just what doctors should do when people want to know whether they should undergo computed tomography to screen for lung cancer or be given vitamins to prevent heart disease. "Sorry," good doctors say, "insufficient evidence."

And this is even truer for children—at least when the question is whether to screen them for early signs or symptoms of adult diseases. First, we need to know whether the problem will even persist into adulthood. Second, do we have a safe and effective treatment? Third and most importantly, does treating the problem in childhood have any effect on clinical outcomes in adulthood?

Which brings us to the case of high blood cholesterol levels—technically, dyslipidemia—in childhood. New guidelines for screening and treatment from the American Academy of Pediatrics have caused a lot of controversy. The pediatricians recommend screening with a fasting lipid profile every 3 to 5 years for all children aged 2 to 10 years who are overweight or have diabetes or a family history of cardiovascular disease. It is reasonable to ask, especially as the epidemic of childhood overweight and obesity has increased the number of children who will be screened, what this screening will accomplish.

---

* "Efficacy" is whether a test or a treatment works in a clinical trial done in a specialized setting; "effectiveness" is whether it works in the real world of everyday care.

Does heart disease start in childhood? It probably does, as autopsies of children who die from other causes have found. And some studies have correlated autopsy findings with dyslipidemia in children. So it would be nice to try to identify children who are at risk of developing heart disease, assuming that we could find them and actually do something that would make a difference when they are adults. But there are a number of problems.

One is that lipid measurement in children is not a perfect marker for present or future heart disease. Lipid concentrations vary during childhood, especially around puberty. They also vary with gender and race. And they don't "track" into adulthood perfectly: somewhere between 30 percent and 50 percent of children with raised cholesterol concentrations won't have them as adults.

A further problem is the treatment for children with raised lipids. Exercise and diet management work, but only in research settings. It's very hard in the real world to get an individual child to eat better, exercise more, and lose weight—and to maintain all of that until adulthood. In addition, as usual, long-term studies that follow such children until they are old enough to have cardiac-related health outcomes are almost impossibly difficult to do.

But the real controversy behind these new guidelines is drug treatment. In a striking departure from previous recommendations, the American Academy of Pediatrics endorses the use from the age of 8 of cholesterol-lowering statin drugs for children who have raised lipid concentrations that have not responded to diet, weight reduction, and exercise. Admittedly this will be a small subset of all children, but commitment to what is likely to be at least 50 years of statin treatment raises many questions.

Do statin medications lower lipid concentrations in children? Yes, they do. Short-term clinical trials of children with familial hypercholesterolemia have found statins to be safe and effective in lowering concentrations of low density lipoprotein (LDL). What about clinical outcomes? As children don't have heart attacks, investigators have looked at the effects of statins on endothelial dysfunction and carotid intimal medial thickness, early markers for atherosclerosis in adults. Controlled studies in children show that, in comparison with control children, statins improve these. So it looks as though statins can make a difference, at least in the short term.

But what about evidence that dozens of years of statin treatment in children with raised lipids will actually improve cardiac outcomes in adulthood? That, of course, is the Holy Grail, and such data are not available. It is likely that they never will be, at least for the foreseeable future. That is a big problem.

I think the obesity epidemic really raises the stakes in this discussion. This is no longer just a discussion of what to do with a very small group of children with an autosomal dominant genetic disorder that virtually guarantees disastrous cardiac outcomes as adults. Now we are moving to mass population screening and treatment of the rapidly increasing number of fat children. Most of them will not have familial hypercholesterolemia, and doctors really don't know what they are doing by treating them for 50 years with statins.

The obesity epidemic is real. We don't have to just stand by and watch it progress. We can and should improve many things, including food and exercise policies in schools, the built environment, and families' diets and physical activity. But I'm very wary of committing a generation of obese children to a lifetime of drug treatment on the basis of pathological markers for possible future disease.

This is preventive medicine, after all. Without good evidence, rather than say, "Don't just stand there—do something," I'd advocate the opposite.

NPR, August 5, 2008

Weighing prostate cancer screening recommendations

The complicated question of whether to screen or not

Prostate cancer screening is in the news again, with new recommendations from the US Preventive Services Task Force. First, a disclosure: I used to work with the task force, and I was the editor of the group's first book 20 years ago. But this discussion is more about the issues behind the prostate cancer screening recommendation than about whether it is right or wrong.

It is important to remember that preventive medicine is optional. When patients come into the office with a broken bone or a burn, doctors have no choice whether to treat them or not. They do the best they can, using whatever information and evidence is available to guide care. That is not the way it is in preventive medicine.

In preventive medicine, everyone wants strong evidence. When you are asking asymptomatic people to come into your office, making them or their insurance company pay for a screening test and exposing them to possible side effects, you had better be clear that what you are doing has been proven to help them.

So—how do you decide whether to get a screening test?

First, you have to know something about the disease you're screening for. It needs to be an important, relatively common and serious disease. We don't screen people for ingrown toenails. But it also helps if the disease has a long asymptomatic phase, when a screening test could find it early. If you get a disease and it is immediately fatal, a screening test won't be of any use.

Second, screening tests all have risks associated with them: side effects, costs, false positives, and so forth. You need one that is affordable, accurate, and has acceptable side effects.

Third and most importantly, screening tests must have proven benefits. They have to identify a previously unknown disease that doctors can actually do something about that makes a difference in health outcomes. And the benefits have to outweigh the harms related both to screening and treatment.

So where does this leave us with prostate cancer screening?

Is prostate cancer a serious, common disease? Absolutely. More than 28,000 American men will die from prostate cancer this year.

Does it progress slowly with a long asymptomatic phase? Yes, it does. Do we have an accurate screening test for it? Well, the blood test called PSA, prostate-specific antigen, is inexpensive and pretty accurate. Its levels do go up with most prostate cancers, although other, more benign things can elevate it, too.

What about the proven benefits of PSA screening? Do they outweigh the harms? This is the problem. There still are no good studies to show that men who get screened and treated for prostate cancer live longer than those who don't. So the benefits are unknown.

The harms of screening and treatment, however, are real and well documented. They include not just the costs and pain of treatment, but also the incontinence and impotence that some men get after surgery. The problem is that some prostate cancer grows quickly and is lethal. Some, especially in older men, is slow-growing and never causes a problem. That is why people say that more older men die *with* prostate cancer than *of* prostate cancer.

Bottom line? Talk to your doctor about these recommendations and pick your screening tests wisely. Make sure that there is good evidence that the benefits outweigh the harms of both diagnosis and treatment.

BMJ, September 6, 2008

Shouting about shots

Why are rates of immunization of children now falling in the US?

One of the (few) things about the US health care "system" that I have always taken pride in is our ability to fully vaccinate nearly all of our children by the time they start school. When I was growing up, before measles vaccine, thousands of cases of measles encephalitis and hundreds of measles-related deaths occurred every year in the United States. By the turn of the present century, though, vaccination programs had eliminated endemic measles, and the few remaining cases were related to travel and immigration.

Not so in Europe. Vaccination coverage is low in several European countries, leading to ongoing outbreaks. And in the United Kingdom in June the Health Protection Agency announced that, because of declining vaccination coverage, measles had again become endemic in England and Wales.

Because it is so contagious, measles is a good harbinger of vaccine coverage. As long as there is measles somewhere in the world, it will be exported by travel and immigration. What happens next depends on immunization rates and resulting coverage. If coverage rates are low, sustained spread of measles takes place. With high coverage, herd immunity* occurs, and imported cases lead only to outbreaks (of varying size) among those who are not vaccinated. Usually they are small and self-limiting, but if sizable pockets of unvaccinated people exists, the outbreaks can be large.

I always felt superior to my British friends and expressed disbelief at the furor in the United Kingdom about possible adverse effects of the measles, mumps, and rubella vaccine. This led to protests, a falling rate of vaccination, and increasingly larger outbreaks. Didn't they get it, I wondered? The threat of endemic measles in a population surely outweighs the disproved or unproved threats of problems caused by vaccine preservatives or the vaccine itself. Something like this would never happen in the US.

---

* The protection afforded all members of a community once a critical proportion of the population is immunized, because there is little opportunity for an outbreak.

But it has. I read with great disappointment a recent Centers for Disease Control and Prevention (CDC) bulletin reporting that the number of measles cases was at a 10-year high in the US in the first half of 2008. It turns out that this spike was not due to an increase in imported cases. Rather, it was attributable to larger numbers of unvaccinated children of school age. The parents of most of them had requested exemptions to school vaccination requirements or had educated their children at home and thus dodged vaccination requirements. The CDC is concerned that these outbreaks may herald a new wave of measles cases around the country.

Although the number of cases, 131, is relatively small, they are crucially important. Some children will always be unvaccinated and vulnerable—all those less than 1 year of age and the small number of older children who are immunologically compromised. They rely on herd immunity for protection. The CDC bulletin says that when the vaccination rate dips below 90 percent in preschool children and below 95 percent in school-age children, herd immunity is no longer as effective, outbreaks get larger, and sustained spread becomes possible.

Almost two-thirds of the unvaccinated children who got measles in the US had not been vaccinated because of their parents' beliefs. And most of these parents were thought to have concerns that the MMR vaccine would cause adverse effects such as autism in their children.

What's going on here? Aren't doctors making it clear to parents what a mistake it is not to vaccinate their children? I don't think that is the problem. Doctors I have spoken to blame much of the parental concern on sensationalist media coverage and the Internet. All you need to do is enter "vaccines and autism" in a search engine to get an eyeful of teary anecdotes and "scientific" correlations claiming to prove the association between shots and disease.

Surely the declining authority of doctors and the increasing impersonality of medical care—and resulting lack of trust—have a role as well. Many people I know are forced to change doctors annually as their health insurance coverage changes. This hinders continuity of care and the growth of a trusting relationship.

Parents may also be rebelling against the seemingly endless number of childhood vaccines that are now recommended. With the addition of rotavirus and pneumococcal vaccines and the return of injections for polio vaccine, it is no surprise that parents express the concern that their children are being turned into pin cushions. If children get shots every month or two from birth to age 18 months, there are plenty of chances to correlate any problems that occur with a recent immunization. If you search hard enough, you can no doubt find that someone somewhere has correlated your child's symptoms—behavioral, neurological, whatever—with a shot that your child has just had.

It's discouraging that real, measurable achievements in public health are in danger of being reversed. I don't have any brilliant suggestions for how to reverse this trend. Government agencies and medical professional societies are doing their best to educate the public about the importance and safety of vaccines. My Internet search brought up many responsible discussions of vaccine safety along with the sob stories and wacko science.

Just as "on the web no one knows you are a dog," it is also true that on the web many will not know you are a charlatan or a well-meaning naïf.

NPR, April 28, 2009

The good news about the flu

Here is what to worry about—and what not to

There is actually a lot of good news about this new swine flu outbreak.

First and foremost, our public health systems—local, state, national, and international—have already found out a lot about the virus. We know that it is a new version of swine flu that has genetic pieces from human, bird, and swine flu viruses. Development of a vaccine to protect people against it is under way. And we know that the swine flu virus is sensitive to some of the antiviral medicines that we have been stockpiling for an occasion such as this.

Second, we have much improved surveillance and communication systems, at least in the US, so that everyone knows what's going on. True, some news outlets are going overboard with scary headlines and ominous music. In general, though, we are getting informative and helpful updates from government agencies of the latest news and advice. I think they have struck just about the right tone of concern but not alarm.

Third, this outbreak is starting late in the winter respiratory infection season, so we will not have a big problem distinguishing swine flu cases from standard flu or other viruses.

Finally, we have learned from 9/11, Katrina, SARS, and the avian flu scare. We are better prepared than ever before to prevent, diagnose, and treat influenza with individual actions, public health measures, antiviral medications, and supportive treatments.

All of which is not to say that we should not be concerned. In the spirit of reassurance, though, here are a few things you do *not* need to worry about.

Some people are making a big deal of the fact that we do not have a longstanding Health and Human Services Secretary or a new Centers for Disease Control and Prevention Director yet in this time of crisis. You don't have to worry about that. There are plenty of capable career employees who know what they're doing minding the store.

On a personal level, you don't need to wear a face mask. You don't have to worry that you didn't get a flu shot last fall; it probably wouldn't have helped much anyway. Finally, you don't have to stay home, keep your kids home, or stay away from other people, unless you're sick.

What should we worry about? That if this infection does spread worldwide we won't have enough medicines and respirators and facilities to take care of everyone. That the virus might increase in severity before we have time to manufacture a lot of vaccine. And that people may panic if and when serious illnesses and deaths start to occur.

Someday, the next worldwide influenza pandemic will strike. This could be it. We are not going to know that for a while. But if it is, and if it is like previous pandemics, it will spread in waves, some mild and some more serious. Either way, we'll be going into it reasonably well prepared.

So, stay calm, get a bottle of hand sanitizer and some tissues to cough or sneeze into. Use them both. Wash your hands with soap or sanitize them before you eat. Don't go to Mexico City if you don't have to. And sit tight.

NPR, November 6, 2009

Does preventive care save money?

What matters is value, not savings

A central question in the debate over the health care overhaul is how to pay for it. Many politicians, including the president, have said that increasing preventive care will save a lot of money in the long term. The Congressional Budget Office, however, has consistently said preventive services will not reduce costs.

Not only do many politicians believe that prevention reduces health care costs, so do most Americans. In a recent survey, 77 percent of Americans agreed that prevention will save us money. It is only logical: find a disease early in its course, treat it, and you not only prevent illness and suffering, but you also save the money you would have spent treating it later.

The problem is that usually it is not literally true. Here's the dirty little secret: most prevention doesn't save money, any more than treatment saves money. The question to ask is not whether preventive medicine saves money, but whether your money is buying good value in health.

A little background. There are three kinds of prevention. Primary prevention takes places before you have a disease and actually prevents it. Childhood immunizations, for example, are the favorite kind of primary prevention. A few shots and you no longer have to worry about your children getting measles or mumps.

Also, counseling people about risky behaviors is primary prevention. If I talk to you about tobacco cessation or sexual behavior and you stop smoking or start using condoms as a result, you're preventing a disease.

Secondary prevention is early detection of an existing disease when it is asymptomatic. Then, you often have a much better chance of curing it. Screening tests are a classic example of secondary prevention. You get a mammogram, find early breast cancer, and get treatment that will, we hope, cure it.

Finally, tertiary prevention is optimal treatment of existing chronic diseases so that you will not develop complications. For instance, patients with diabetes need regular eye and foot exams to watch out for retinal problems and foot ulcers.

It turns out that some preventive medicine actually does save money. For example, the cost of vaccinating an entire population against some diseases is less than it would have cost to treat those diseases if they developed in some of the people. Most types of prevention, however, do not literally save money. The reason for this is that you have to screen a lot of women with mammography, for example, in order to find one breast cancer.

So, if it does not save money, how do we decide what prevention is worth doing? That is where value comes in.

As Steven Woolf and others argued in a recent paper on this subject, the question of whether prevention saves money and thus can help pay for health care reform misses the point. What does matter, and this matters both for prevention and treatment services, is value—the health benefit per dollar invested.

Preventive services are worth it if they improve health at a relatively low cost. The way we control health care spending is by moving our money from expensive, low-value services—both treatment and prevention—to more cost-effective, but not necessarily cost-saving, high-value interventions. That means fewer expensive drugs that extend life a week or a month, and more proven early interventions that can extend life for years or decades.

Yes, prevention does not save money, but effective preventive care, like effective treatment, will be a crucial part of a reformed health care system.

NPR, October 13, 2009

Debate over the H1N1 vaccine? There shouldn't be one

Myths about the new swine flu vaccine

Public health authorities at the federal, state, and local levels are clear in their recommendations: virtually everyone should get a pandemic flu shot, with precedence given to those at increased risk of infection and complications.

First in line to get the vaccine are pregnant women and those who live with or take care of children younger than 6 months of age (they are too young to be vaccinated). Then come health care and emergency services workers and young people from 6 months to 24 years old. Add people who are older than 24 with diabetes, asthma, or other diseases that make them high risk. Finally, the lowest priority goes to all of us healthy middle-aged and older people, who may already have some immunity to this flu virus.

Given these straightforward recommendations, why would you not want to get the vaccine? People under age 50 have no immunity to this virus, which means it is very infectious.

First possible concern: the new vaccine isn't safe. People say it hasn't been tested enough, they rushed to make it too quickly, and I don't want to be a guinea pig.

Wrong.

This new vaccine was made the same way, with the same ingredients, and at the same factories as regular seasonal flu vaccine, which is an extremely safe vaccine. There has been no evidence of harm or serious side effects in the vaccine trials that were conducted, and the worst you can expect from the vaccine is a sore arm for a day or two.

Second concern: Why get the vaccine when everyone says the pandemic flu is a mild disease: a few days, a little cough and fever? I probably won't get it anyway.

Wrong and wrong.

While it is true that most people who have gotten the disease have not become seriously ill, people under age 50 have no immunity to this virus, which means it is very infectious. When you have a lot of people infected—

and we're talking potentially tens of millions here—some of them are going to get very sick, get hospitalized, and even die. It has happened in many states already: young, previously healthy men and especially pregnant women have died from this strain of pandemic influenza. That is big news.

Related to the last concern is the opinion that there is no need to get the vaccine because you can just take one of the antiviral medicines to treat your flu if it gets bad.

Wrong.

While it is true that so far we have antiviral medicines that are effective treatments for pandemic flu, they need to be reserved for severe cases or for people who are at increased risk of becoming very ill, like those with asthma. If everyone starts using antiviral medicines, the flu virus will likely mutate to become resistant to the medicines and we are in big trouble.

Finally, some people say they can't afford the new vaccine, especially if they have already paid for the regular, seasonal flu vaccine.

Wrong.

You have already paid for the vaccine with your taxes. The federal government has bought all the vaccine and is giving it away. The most you will pay is an administration fee, and many people will pay nothing at all.

Bottom line? The pandemic flu vaccine is safe, effective, cheap or free, and necessary. Unless you're allergic to eggs, when it becomes available in your area, make sure you get it, and make especially sure that your kids do, too.

BMJ, December 5, 2009

Mammograms, poor communication, and politics

What lessons can be learned from the furor over new breast screening recommendations?

The US Preventive Services Task Force, though appointed and staffed by the government, is an independent, rotating panel of doctors, nurses, and methodologists. Its mission since 1984 has been to systematically review the evidence on clinical preventive services—screening tests, chemoprevention agents, and counseling interventions—and to publish recommendations based on their findings. (Full disclosure: I formerly directed the task force staff and edited its first book in 1989.)

The task force is no stranger to controversy. In order to recommend a given preventive service, its methodology requires good evidence that the benefits exceed the harms. Many of the panel's early recommendations, when systematic reviews and evidence-based recommendations were not widespread, differed from those of established authorities. Disease-specific advocacy groups and medical specialty societies were often furious when the task force did not agree with them about the effectiveness of various screening tests for colorectal, prostate, skin, or breast cancer or for lead poisoning or coronary artery disease.

Relations between the task force and other groups have generally been better since the late 1990s, because evidence-based methods have become mainstream, and in some cases (such as for colorectal cancer) new trials have been published that allowed the task force to broaden its recommendations. Also, the task force became better known in the United States and more prestigious. It was officially authorized by Congress and its recommendations were cited in legislation concerning the Medicare program and preventive services. Current health reform proposals refer to services recommended by the task force in mandating appropriate preventive care. As a result of these trends, recommendations of specialty societies, advocacy groups, and the task force have in many cases become similar, if not identical.

Breast cancer screening seemed to be an example of this trend when, in 2002, the task force changed its longstanding neutral ("C") ranking of mammography for women in their 40s to a positive one, recommending screening every 1 to 2 years for women aged 40 or older. This was similar to recommendations from groups such as the American Cancer Society and the American College of Obstetricians and Gynecologists.

So it should have been no surprise that, when the task force seemingly reversed its 2002 position on November 17 this year, recommending against routine screening of women in their 40s, it would make headlines. In fact it unleashed a firestorm. The story made the front pages of national newspapers daily for most of the week. The recommendations were widely and loudly denounced by radiologists, breast cancer survivors, media doctors, gynecologists, and politicians. Medical experts called the task force "idiots," and conservatives lined up to denounce the report as an Obama administration plot foreshadowing what would happen under health reform.

What in the world happened? Almost no one disagrees about the evidence. Screening mammography can save women's lives if it is started in their 40s, but it is much more accurate in older than younger women. The task force reviewed the number needed to screen to prevent one breast cancer death, which is around 1,900 women in their 40s versus 377 women in their 60s. It looked at six new modeling studies, which found that an average of 80 percent of the effectiveness of breast cancer screening could be achieved with screenings every 2 years, averting almost half of the false positives. It considered the rising number of mammography-induced overdiagnoses—cancers that either would not have progressed or for which early discovery and treatment conferred no benefit. Then, fatefully, it changed its recommendation for women in their 40s back to a C rating and increased the recommended screening interval for older women to every two years.

The panel's intent in this change was to recommend that women in their 40s discuss the benefits and harms of screening with their doctors. The language accompanying the new recommendation is virtually identical to that in the 2002 advice. But because of a redefinition of the C rating that had taken place after the 2002 report, this rating now has negative rather than neutral language associated with it. As a result, the headlines screamed that it was a recommendation against mammography for women in their 40s.

Thus, misleading wording was directed at a touchstone and emblematic issue. It was introduced into the present supercharged political climate in the US in which every health issue is reflected through the prism of health reform and the budget. In short, they hit the trifecta. It is no wonder that a furor was the result.

The potential damage of this poorly timed and worded report is surprisingly large. Many women are confused and upset. The task force is discredited and even endangered. The Agency for Healthcare Research and Quality, which sponsors the task force, is threatened and has distanced itself from the task force. By extension, perhaps the entire health reform effort is damaged. It is a stunning development.

Lessons learned? This fiasco may not have been preventable, but a better appreciation of the politics of breast cancer and of health reform might have helped. More careful wordsmithing and timing was certainly called for. Overall, it is a stinging lesson about the surprising importance and potentially devastating consequences of changing an arcane definition of an obscure rating system used by a prominent scientific advisory panel.

BMJ, March 13, 2010

Is hypertension really a neglected disease?

If the Institute of Medicine says so, it must be true

Quick, what do you think of when you hear the term "neglected disease"? Kala-azar, perhaps, or schistosomiasis? Me, too. In fact, Wikipedia, the source of all knowledge these days, says that the neglected diseases are "a group of tropical infections which are especially endemic in low-income populations in developing regions of Africa, Asia, and the Americas." So I was a little surprised to read a new US Institute of Medicine (IOM) report that says that hypertension should be added to the list of neglected diseases.

Everyone knows the IOM. Usually termed the "prestigious Institute of Medicine," it is the most junior branch of the US National Academies, "advisers to the nation on science, engineering, and medicine" (as their tagline has it). IOM, chartered in 1970, includes about 1,200 distinguished medical doctors and scientists. They serve on various committees and issue reports on all manner of health-related topics at the request of the government and foundations.

The Centers for Disease Control and Prevention (CDC), specifically its division for heart disease and stroke prevention, commissioned this report. The CDC asked IOM for guidance on what its role should be in reducing and controlling high blood pressure. A committee was assembled, they and IOM staff worked on it for a year, and they have just issued their findings and recommendations.

Interestingly, just about their first conclusion was that—wait for it— given the burden of disease represented by hypertension, CDC's program is "dramatically underfunded." This is pretty standard stuff in IOM reports. Agency asks (and pays) for guidance, IOM looks into it, and two findings emerge: the problem is really big and important, and the requesting agency needs more funds to fight it. CDC has always been a poor sister to the National Institutes of Health. The National Heart, Lung, and Blood Institute gets a cool $3 billion a year, compared with a paltry $54 million for CDC's heart disease prevention division. Are you listening, Congress?

To be fair, there is a lot more to the report.

It begins by laying out the magnitude of the problem. Hypertension is common, affecting almost a third of all American adults. After decreasing from about 1970 to 1990, the prevalence of hypertension has risen in the past two decades. It is one of the leading causes of death, accounting for about 45 percent of all cardiovascular deaths. And it is expensive, with direct and indirect costs estimated to exceed $73 billion a year in the United States. Hypertension is highly treatable, often with inexpensive, generic drugs, together with weight loss, proper diet, and exercise. It is even, in many cases, preventable, through the same hygienic measures.

Despite the relative ease of treatment and the wide attention it has had through such initiatives as the National High Blood Pressure Education Program, hypertension is not well controlled in many patients. Although more than 70 percent of people with hypertension are aware of their condition, only 61 percent are treated, and only 35 percent are under good control.

The reasons for this are not well understood. Some of it is due to access and economic factors, some is patients' attitudes and knowledge, and some is lack of proper treatment by doctors. Long-discredited ideas, such as the benign nature of isolated systolic hypertension,* still have a hold on many doctors. Some doctors won't treat "mildly" elevated blood pressure or will allow elderly patients "10 points per decade" over 60 before they consider treatment. This is where the neglect comes in, I guess. Patients know they are hypertensive. Doctors know they are hypertensive. Too little gets done about it.

The report recommends that, given CDC's limited resources, public health interventions will deliver more bang for the buck than one-on-one clinical treatment. The problems with the public health approach, however, are obvious. First, interventions are easy to list but hard to implement. How does a government agency spend money wisely to decrease a population's obesity, increase physical activity, and encourage heart-healthy diets? Second, with one exception, there is nothing unique to hypertension about these interventions. They are the same ones recommended for preventing obesity, diabetes, arthritis, and almost everything else that ails us. Only

---

* When the top number—the systolic pressure—in a blood pressure reading is elevated while the bottom number—diastolic pressure—remains normal. Example: 165/70.

sodium reduction is particular to high blood pressure. That might be one of the public health take-home messages from this report, if we can figure out population strategies to decrease salt consumption.

Even though the report focuses on population-based policies and system changes, I am still drawn to the clinical challenge. The day the report came out I asked some family medicine residents if they thought hypertension was a "neglected" disease. They looked at me as though I were nuts. "We spend all day every day treating high blood pressure." That's what I thought, too, but just for fun we pulled some patient charts at random. A surprising number had blood pressures above 140/90 mm Hg, despite being "under treatment."

So maybe my cynicism was uncalled for. Maybe hypertension is indeed a neglected disease. Maybe I should add it to my short list of things we doctors have to do well in order to be members of the Good Doctors' Club. And maybe this IOM report is an important one after all.

BMJ, October 9, 2010

Depressed about depression

Depression is common and important, but are public screening days the answer?

The Centers for Disease Control and Prevention (CDC) has just published 2006 and 2008 state-based population rates for current depression in the United States. Using seven questions from the Patient Health Questionnaire-8 (PHQ-8) depression screening tool, which have been incorporated into their telephone-administered Behavioral Risk Factor Surveillance System Survey, they found that 9 percent of the respondents met criteria for current depression (present in the previous 2 weeks). This included 3.4 percent who met the criteria for major depression. The sample size for this survey is very large—more than 235,000—but the response rates can be low, varying by state from 37 percent to 73 percent.

These data were released by the CDC with an advertisement for and to coincide with National Depression Screening Day, an annual event that takes place every fall in the US during a larger program called Mental Illness Awareness Week. More about this shortly.

As the new data from CDC confirm yet again, depression is common. It is important as well. Everyone knows that the suicide rate is higher among depressed people and that a high proportion (up to half) of patients who kill themselves are depressed. Many are not aware, however, of the huge toll that depression takes on people who are not suicidal. It is estimated that by 2020, major depression will be second only to heart disease as the leading cause of disability. Major depression is not just the blues. It has huge personal, social, and economic implications.

Depression is treatable. Drugs or talk therapy (or both), with good follow-up, can reliably decrease symptoms and disability in around half of those with major depression. New treatment guidelines have just been issued by the American Psychiatric Association. Despite this, many people with depression remain untreated. Some are unaware of their disease and don't seek help. Some manifest it through somatic* symptoms and thus the depression itself is not diagnosed. Some are ashamed or embarrassed to discuss "feelings." Primary care doctors often fail to recognize many patients with depression, for all these reasons as well as lack of training.

Given the above, it would seem logical that we should screen in primary care to find undetected depression and treat it. Twenty-five years ago I worked at the National Institute for Mental Health in a small primary care research program, and this was an interest of ours. At that time there was no good evidence that screening for depression in primary care would actually lead to improved outcomes among patients. The first report of the US Preventive Services Task Force (USPSTF), in 1989, reflected this and did not recommend routine screening for depression in primary care.

Since then, however, research has shown that screening for depression in primary care is effective. By 2002, the USPSTF was recommending routine screening, as long as practices had systems in place to ensure accurate diagnosis, effective treatment, and follow-up care. This was an important caveat. Many studies found little or no improvement after simple screening and feedback of results; only when there was a planned path of screening, feedback, treatment, and follow-up were consistently positive results found. Last year the task force updated its recommendation with more specificity, stipulating that "staff-assisted depression care supports" also needed to be in place. Again, a systematic review of current research showed much less benefit without onsite staff whose job it was to guide patients into care and follow them up periodically.

All of which brings us back to National Depression Screening Day, when depression screening is offered to the public in hundreds of health care facilities, health fairs, shopping malls, and workplaces around the US. On the screening day, clinicians volunteer their time to offer free depression screening and information sessions to anyone who wishes to drop in.

The program's website says that those attending will be able to complete a written screening questionnaire, discuss results with a health professional, receive a referral list of local treatment options, watch an educational video, pick up pamphlets and brochures, and fill in a questionnaire for a loved one. Last year more than 1,000 depression screening events were held across the country.

---

* Physical symptoms, such as pain, fatigue, poor appetite, or weight loss.

Not to be a grinch, but where is the evidence that this type of activity makes any difference at all? Screening for health problems at health fairs and such is largely a worthless endeavor, mainly identifying people who already know they have a problem (such as hypertension or hypercholesterolemia) and generally failing to supply follow up or even referrals for ongoing care and evaluation. Since Don Berwick first wrote about this 25 years ago, mass screening at health fairs has remained unproved and largely discredited.

The depression screening day has slightly more going for it than health fairs, but it is a much more difficult disease to diagnose and treat than hypertension or high cholesterol. Even if clinicians supervise the screening test and discuss the results, will they or their offices ensure that the possibly depressed patients get a proper diagnosis, treatment, and follow-up? I think not. It is great to inform the world about depression. It is a terribly important problem that has real consequences and proven treatments. But screening people at 1-day themed events, let alone on the web, strikes me as both a waste of everyone's time and a misleading promise of diagnosis and treatment that probably won't be delivered.

BMJ, November 20, 2010

Screening for early detection of lung cancer

At long last, something that makes a difference?

I give an annual lecture to first year medical students on what makes a good screening test. One of the hardest points to get across is that early detection does not necessarily lead to improved outcomes. Why isn't it the case, they ask, that finding cancer early is not always better than finding it later? It is so counterintuitive.

To answer I cite the randomized controlled trials (RCTs) done in the 1970s that tested chest X-rays and sputum cytology as screening tests for lung cancer. Despite the fact that the screening tests found many asymptomatic lung cancers, none of the trials decreased mortality rates among the smokers who were screened, in comparison with controls. We would never have known this without RCTs, given that early detection nicely increased "survival times." Really what was increasing was just the length of time that patients knew they had the disease.

RCTs have always been seen as the gold standard in evaluating screening tests because they eliminate many of the biases that taint uncontrolled observational studies. As a result of the RCTs of lung cancer screening, it was with some confidence that the US Preventive Services Task Force and other evidence-based authorities recommended against using chest radiography to screen for lung cancer. As opposed to many other preventive services, here we had direct evidence on whether a screening test worked or not. Plus, a more recent analysis of a huge screening trial for prostate, lung, and colorectal cancer has confirmed that screening chest X-rays don't effectively reduce lung cancer mortality.

But lung cancer remains a critical problem. It is the leading cause of cancer deaths among men and (since they started smoking more) women. It is estimated that more than 157,000 Americans will die from lung cancer this year. It kills more people each year than do cancers of the breast, prostate, and colon *combined*. Unlike survival from most other cancers, lung cancer survival has seen no significant improvement over the past 30 years. Up to 85 percent of patients with lung cancer die from their disease.

The good news is that this may be about to change.

On November 4, the National Cancer Institute announced that it had terminated its National Lung Screening Trial (NLST) early because of positive results. The number of deaths from lung cancer was 20 percent lower among heavy smokers who were screened annually three times with low-dose helical computed tomography (CT) than among those screened with conventional chest radiography. This RCT was huge news, making the front pages of national newspapers despite being released just two days after our elections.

Hints about the effectiveness of CT screening for lung cancer have been appearing over the past 10 years, during which several single-arm* CT screening studies were published. Although their study designs did not permit a reliable assessment of the effect of the screening on cancer mortality, it was clearly a promising technology. CT's cross-sectional views reduce the problem of overlying structures obscuring details, which plagues regular chest X-rays. Their improved contrast allows more subtle abnormalities to be identified. Treatments may have improved in recent years as well, although patients in the NLST trial did not get specialized care; they were referred for routine treatment once their cancers were diagnosed.

To their credit, everyone connected with the press release was careful to add caveats to the big news. This was just a preliminary press report, they said. The final analyses had not yet been done, let alone published in peer-reviewed journals. The study applied only to heavy (30 or more packs a year) smokers aged 55 or older. And it seemed to be required to add that smoking cessation is still the most effective and proven way to prevent lung cancer. How refreshing!

There are indeed plenty of questions left to ask. Around a quarter of the patients enrolled in the trial had a positive scan result, the vast majority of which were false positives. Given that heavy smokers will have all kinds of noncancerous changes in their lungs that will be picked up by CT, the costs of screening in terms of worry, follow-up testing, and side effects will be high. At up to $300 a scan, the dollar costs will be high as well.

Then there is the radiation exposure. Though they produce only 25 percent of the radiation of a diagnostic scan, low-dose CT scanning

---

* Trials without a control group, or "arm."

still emits much more ionizing radiation than regular X-rays. What is the cumulative radiation risk of 7, or 10, or 20 annual scans?

On the other hand, the efficacy of screening CT for lung cancer may be even greater than the 20 percent announced last week. The study was stopped early. Longer follow-up would likely have allowed time for more deaths in the control group, increasing the benefit of the CTs. Also, the study provided only three annual scans. What would have happened if more scans were done? Finally, there is the matter of all-cause mortality, which was reduced by 7 percent in the CT group. No one knows for sure why that happened, but it may be a side-benefit as well.

Many of these questions will be answered soon when the formal analyses of the trial are published. Others will have to await longer follow-up. Still others will remain unanswered. No matter how you look at it, however, it is great news indeed to have even a preliminary report of a large, well-conducted RCT of a screening test for the leading cause of cancer deaths that led to a significant reduction in mortality.

BMJ, June 11, 2011

AIDS at 30: A chance to treat is a chance to prevent

The question for tomorrow is how to pay for it

Thirty years ago, on June 4, 1981, the CDC published a small case series of previously healthy homosexual men in Los Angeles who had contracted pneumocystis pneumonia. A month later, 26 more cases were described, from New York as well as California, and some of them had Kaposi's sarcoma, another disease seen most commonly in immune-compromised patient.

So it began.

Gay men were the initial focus, but then hemophiliacs and others receiving transfusions and injection drug users were stricken. Stricken was the appropriate word. Almost everyone with AIDS in the early days died, and most died within months of the appearance of symptoms. Drugs commonly used to treat their infections and cancers didn't work. Many of the deaths were horrible: pneumonia, complicated by intractable diarrhea, severe mouth ulcers, skin lesions, and more. I took care of a few early AIDS patients during my residency, and it was awful and frustrating for them, their loved ones, and their doctors and nurses.

It is stunning to look back and realize that in 30 years, more than 60 million people have been infected with HIV, and at least half of them have died from it.

In context, the medical reaction to the epidemic was remarkably rapid, but it seemed very slow at the time. In 1983, HIV was discovered, and the next year it was proved to cause AIDS. By 1985, we had a diagnostic test for HIV, so infections could be discovered in much earlier stages.

No treatment was available then, but the modes of transmission were clear and behavioral change in at-risk populations became the prevention strategy of choice. Activists in the gay community led the fight for behavior changes as well as demanding more funding for research, speedier drug trials and licensing, and increased participation by patients and their caregivers.

In a recent reminiscence, Anthony Fauci, then (as now) leading NIH research on AIDS, recalls being "vilified" by AIDS activists for not moving fast enough to address the crisis. As a minor government functionary in the mid- and late 1980s, I watched the drama unfold, attending coordinating meetings led by Fauci while pickets marched outside our building. Everyone was trying hard, but people were dying horrible deaths as the clock ticked on.

In 1987, zidovudine (then called AZT) was licensed, and finally we had a drug that would help. Lives were prolonged, and some patients did very well indeed. The early drugs were toxic, though, and they had to be taken many times a day on a very demanding schedule.

Almost 25 years after zidovudine, we have come a long way. Dozens of antiretroviral drugs are now in use, and their side effects and dosage regimens are much more tolerable. Many patients can take a single combination capsule once or twice a day. When treated appropriately, life expectancy has increased from 6 *months* from the emergence of clinical symptoms 30 years ago to perhaps 50 *years* today, when measured from the initial diagnosis of asymptomatic HIV infection. HIV infection has changed from being a death sentence to a disease managed like many other complex conditions: routine appointments in primary care combined with regular consultations with specialists.

To complement treatment we also now have a large collection of proven prevention strategies in addition to abstinence and condoms: needle exchange for injection drug users, post-exposure prophylaxis for medical personnel, maternal drug treatment to prevent transmission to newborns, blood bank testing to prevent transfusion-associated cases, and circumcision and topical gels to prevent transmission to women.

These are crucial, because we are still seeing two to three new infections emerge for every person put on lifesaving treatment. Worldwide, it is estimated that there were 2.6 million new infections in 2009. Ninety percent of people with AIDS are living in developing countries. Huge progress has been made in providing antiretroviral treatment for millions of them, through the generosity of large charities and Western governments. Some 85 percent of antiretroviral treatment in the developing world, at a cost of $8.3 billion, was provided from these sources.

Much more still needs to be done, though. This is especially true since the treatment and prevention worlds have now merged, with the dramatic announcement last month of the early results of NIH's HPTN 052 trial. This randomized controlled trial, largely among heterosexual couples in the developing world, found that early *treatment* of HIV dramatically decreased *transmission* of the virus to regular sexual partners. As long suspected from observational data, the best prevention turns out also to be early and effective treatment.

Prices for antiretroviral drugs in the developing world have dramatically decreased due to the availability of inexpensive generic drugs. Even so, in light of the results from the NIH trial, the potential costs for treating all infected patients, while maintaining other prevention programs and research, is likely to be staggering. NIH scientists are modeling what it would cost to treat everyone, and how various strategies would affect transmission and thus the emergence of future new cases. The costs will likely be in the hundreds of billions of dollars.

The challenge confronting us soon will be how to find the resources to treat everyone (or almost everyone) in order to slow the growth of new cases and write the final chapter of the AIDS story.

3

Politics, Health, and Health Care

"The health of the people is really the foundation upon which all their happiness and all their powers as a state depend."
—Benjamin Disraeli, 1804–1881

It is no surprise that this section contains the largest number of essays in the book. Health and health care are inevitably intertwined with politics, for two reasons: money and ideology.

As the annual bill for health care in the US has soared into multiple trillions of dollars, it has become both a big business and a budgetary nightmare. As a result, everything related to health is now viewed through the prism of costs, and everyone is in the business of delivering cost-effective care—if we can just figure out what that is.

Political (as well as religious) ideology also affects how people see health and health care. Is there a right to health care? Should we allocate resources to cover the entire population, or focus on paying for unlimited care for older Americans? Are condoms a way to prevent pregnancy and disease or a moral abomination? The answers all depend on what you believe.

When Pope Benedict XVI gave an interview on his way to Africa that seemed to dismiss the effectiveness of condoms in preventing the spread of HIV and other diseases, the public health community was in an uproar. I wrote a column calling for a compromise solution—permitting condom use for disease prevention purposes, if not for contraception. Subsequently there was a hint that the Catholic Church might just consider such an option.

During the election campaign of 2008, I searched the health platforms of all the major candidates—Democrats and Republicans—looking in vain for a plank supporting the importance and central role of primary care medicine in a reformed health care system. I couldn't find it anywhere, so I wrote a column about it. Similarly, none of the candidates had pledged to reverse the Bush administration's blatantly political distortion of politically inconvenient scientific and medical research findings. I thought that deserved mention as well. Finally, there were several instances in which the US surgeon general was muzzled for trying to give scientifically sound public health advice. That, and what I considered to be the wrong-headed criteria being used to select a new surgeon general, also led to commentaries.

Prominent individuals also play a role in the politics of health care, of course, and I have profiled three of them in separate commentaries. Elizabeth Edwards, sadly now deceased, first came to public attention as the wife of a senator and presidential candidate, but then became a political figure in her own right as she battled cancer in a very public way. Thomas Daschle, a former senator and consummate political insider, was odds-on favorite to become President Obama's health secretary before he withdrew because of financial improprieties. Donald Berwick, an internationally respected pediatrician and health quality guru, has been pilloried inappropriately for promoting—gasp—rationing of health care, as he serves a congressionally shortened term running the US Medicare program. All of their stories provide interesting lessons in the politics of health care.

This section also focuses on major public health issues. Tobacco remains the leading cause of death in the US, but funds to help decrease tobacco use are being crowded out by an even more urgent epidemic, obesity. I wrote about whether or not this should be an either-or situation. A great example of the influence of political pressure on public health is the saga of taxes on sugar-sweetened beverages. I told the story of how the strong intervention of the beverage industry stopped an almost sure-fire way to help slow the obesity epidemic. Finally, some people do not consider gun control to be a public health issue. I think that when demonstrably mentally ill persons have ready access to semiautomatic weapons with high-capacity bullet clips, something needs to be done.

These many discussions about what the best public health approaches are for improving health status, however, may all be for naught. Look at the first essay I wrote for the *BMJ*, in 2007, which begins this section. In it I bemoaned that fact that much of what doctors do, and even most of what the health system does, pale in comparison to the individual attribute that has the strongest correlation with longevity: years of education.

BMJ, January 20, 2007

Today's doctors' dilemma

The secret to a longer life is nothing we can do anything about in health care

To George Bernard Shaw in his play *The Doctor's Dilemma*, the dilemma doctors faced was choosing between helping patients and helping themselves to lucrative fees. Today's doctors' dilemma is that what we do doesn't make much difference.

As a young man disillusioned by the politics of the late 1960s, I sought refuge in medicine. I thought that the government and politics were making things worse. The only hope I saw was helping one patient at a time. I would work as a family doctor, my patients would feel better, and thus I would make the world a better place. The answer was medical.

I was wrong. After working in a health center in an economically deprived neighborhood only a short time, even I figured out that I couldn't "fix" much of what was wrong with my patients. Sure, I could prescribe pills and insulin for my diabetic patients, but many of them had neither the means to buy healthy foods nor access to well-stocked stores from which to purchase them. I could refer patients to dietitians to learn about healthy eating, but many couldn't read the leaflets they were given. I could immunize children against an increasing number of illnesses, but many fell victim to epidemics we didn't have shots to prevent: drugs, tobacco, and violence. The answer was societal, not medical.

Twenty years later, Michael McGinnis and William Foege published data showing that the leading causes of death in the United States were not the heart disease, cancers, and strokes I was treating. Medically, we knew what to do about them. Instead, tobacco, bad diet, physical inactivity, and alcohol were actually what was killing people. This was an unconventional conclusion, even among public health types. I certainly hadn't spent much time learning about any of these problems in medical school or residency. The answer must be preventive medicine. Knowing what the problems are and doing something about them are two different things, however.

Ten years later, America is still doing a rotten job of delivering preventive care. The Agency for Healthcare Research and Quality has just published its annual *National Healthcare Quality Report*. Their conclusion? "The use of proven prevention strategies lags significantly behind other gains in health care." Only half of adults over 50 get screened for colorectal cancer. A third of smokers don't receive advice to quit. Less than 60 percent of elderly people have ever had pneumococcal vaccine. Twenty percent of children under the age of 3 have not received all recommended immunizations.

One solution to this problem is to pay doctors to do preventive care. The current experience in the United Kingdom's National Health Service is instructive here. Shaw would have loved learning that at least some of today's British general practitioners are getting rich not by doing unneeded surgeries but by doing thousands of Pap smears and flu shots. The US Medicare program says doctors will soon be able to increase their reimbursement also if they deliver better care to the elderly, some of which will no doubt be defined as more preventive care.

But we have a long way to go. In America we are much more interested in finding the next new blockbuster (or even "me-too") drug than in what Steven Woolf calls "fidelity of existing interventions." We spend billions of dollars inventing and testing new drugs that only marginally extend the benefits of those they replace, rather than putting resources into better delivery of existing effective services. Woolf and his colleague Robert Johnson have shown, for example, that heroic searches for better cholesterol-lowering and antiplatelet drugs cost more and result in less population health gain than would the delivery of today's statins and aspirin to all those who could benefit from them.

Much of this is not rocket science. If there is a budget for it, we can improve health care quality, including the quality of preventive care, with known tools: evidence-based guidelines, reminder systems, computerized physician order entry systems, and electronic medical records. It would be nice if future years' national quality reports found great leaps of progress rather than what they admit are now only modest and uneven gains. This must be the answer.

But it is not. What is the single factor that best predicts longevity? It is not smoking, diet, or receipt of appropriate preventive care. It is not race or wealth. Recently, British GP Iona Heath argued elegantly that we should focus on treating the sick rather than treating risk factors that we have turned into diseases; but that too would have little or no effect on lifespan. In fact, the secret to a longer life is nothing we can do anything about in health care.

That is today's doctors' dilemma. It is not the conflict between what is good for our patients and what is good for our pocketbook. It is not choosing between sickness care and prevention, or between medical care and public health services. Most authorities are now convinced that education—years in school—has the most direct causal effect on how long people live. We can work around the margins with our statins and nicotine replacement patches and mammograms. We can relieve suffering and tend to the sick. But for every extra year spent in school, life expectancy is extended 18 months. Even bleeding heart liberals like me don't think that it is a doctor's job to get kids to stay in school.

BMJ, April 14, 2007

The cancer diagnosis that has gripped America

The unpredictability of cancer may help explain media obsession with a presidential candidate's wife

I have been surprised by the extensive and continuing media coverage of the announcement that Elizabeth Edwards, wife of the US presidential candidate John Edwards, has recurrent breast cancer. It was front page news when it was announced. The Edwards's decision to continue his campaign despite the cancer was then analyzed and discussed endlessly, with multiple follow-up stories and interviews in the newspapers, on the network news programs, and in the blogosphere. Why all the fuss?

First, a bit of background. John Edwards, a former US senator, ran for president in 2004 and was beaten by John Kerry, who then picked him as his vice presidential running mate. On election day 2004, Mrs. Edwards found out that she had breast cancer. She subsequently had surgery and radiation therapy and was pronounced cured. John Edwards is running again for president in the 2008 election and generally has been third in public opinion polls, after Hillary Rodham Clinton and Barack Obama.

Further relevant background. The Edwardses had two teenage children. Their 16-year-old son died in 1996 in a car crash. In her late 40s Elizabeth Edwards then had two more children, who are now aged 6 and 8.

On March 22, Elizabeth and John Edwards held a press conference to announce that her breast cancer had returned. It has metastasized to her bones and possibly to internal organs as well. Although the cancer is stage IV and incurable, her cancer burden is small, and her doctors told her that it is "completely treatable." She said that she feels well, is planning to undergo unspecified treatments to control her cancer, and that she and her husband had jointly decided to press on with his campaign.

The pundits are having a field day with this one. Elizabeth and John Edwards were immediately called courageous and forthright by many, but others have criticized their decision to carry on with the campaign under such uncertain circumstances. Some thought it callous to focus on his career instead of her health. Others say that they are short-changing their young children by not spending every possible minute with them. Katie Couric, the television network news anchor who famously lost her own husband to colon cancer, interviewed them and asked whether they were in denial and being unrealistic in their expectations. Many wondered how candidate (let alone President) Edwards could focus on the affairs of the world while his wife's health is so precarious. Others saw this as a plea for a sympathy vote.

Mrs. Edwards responded by saying that all of us are dying; her only difference is that she now knows what she will die from. She wants to be seen as living with cancer rather than dying from it, and to her the only choice is whether to "push forward or start dying." She and her husband have spoken about their young children and how they told them the news. John Edwards says that he wants no one to vote for him out of sympathy but that voters may learn something important about him from this. He feels that he has shown his ability to continue to function in his job during periods of family stress because he has done it twice before: when their elder son died and at the time of his wife's first cancer diagnosis.

So why all the press furor over this news? I think there are three reasons. First, Americans are obsessed with the domestic affairs of our political leaders. Nothing that Hillary Rodham Clinton does as a candidate for president engenders greater interest and attention than her role as wronged wife during her husband's presidency. Similarly, the Republican candidate Rudy Giuliani, former mayor of New York, gets more press for the ongoing saga of his wives and their previous husbands than for his policy statements. John Edwards only made it onto the daily network news shows when his wife's cancer recurrence was revealed.

Second, this was a recurrence of cancer, not a primary diagnosis. As one of my friends, herself a cancer survivor, said, "Everyone's got breast cancer—it's no big deal." It is commonplace to hear about a celebrity with breast cancer who undergoes treatment and announces that she is cured. Recurrence, however, is not part of the public drill. It is scarier, and terms such as "stage IV," "metastases," and "incurable" upset the press and the public. In a world full of media consultants and carefully scripted appearances, everyone understands that the future for this couple is not predictable. It is going to play out in real time in front of the entire country.

Finally, and related to that, there is clearly something very special about Elizabeth Edwards. Her direct, no-nonsense approach is genuine and appealing. Her intelligence, thoughtfulness, and toughness come through clearly. She is a woman who has been given much but has also been put through much. We all wonder how we would deal with such devastating news in private and in public. At least some of us, myself included, would hope for her strength and grace. It is as much about us as them.

As actor Tim Robbins's character Andy Dufresne said in the film *The Shawshank Redemption*, "It usually comes down to a simple choice, really: get busy living or get busy dying."

BMJ, August 18, 2007

Conflicts in office

A former surgeon general's testimony reveals battles between science and politics

In a July congressional hearing, the immediate past US surgeon general, Richard Carmona, testified about the problem of political meddling in what he saw as the proper functions and activities of his office.

Carmona spoke generally about repeated interference by the George W. Bush administration (which appointed him) in his attempts to speak out on controversial issues, such as stem cell research, abstinence-only sex education, and the emergency contraceptive pill. His speeches were scrubbed of any mention of these matters, even when his comments were based on science.

The former surgeon general also said that he was told by an unnamed senior Bush administration official that he didn't "get it" when it came to the political basis for scientific reports, which had to agree with the administration's political agenda or they would not be approved. Two other former surgeons general—C. Everett Koop, from the Reagan years, and David Satcher, from the Clinton presidency—also testified and cited similar examples from their own tenures. They said, however, that the censorship seemed to be getting worse.

The testimony brought a swift response from the Bush administration and from Washington's punditocracy. The administration dismissed Carmona's charges, saying that it had given him all the support and opportunities he needed and that it was disappointing "if he failed to use his position to the fullest extent." The pundits either praised him for coming forward with his story or questioned his courage for waiting until he had left office before speaking out.

Carmona's general accusations became more specific at the end of July, when the *Washington Post* said in a front page story that one of the reports Carmona was complaining about was a 2006 global health study. It was never released, because Carmona would not make political changes demanded by a Bush official named William Steiger. A godson of the first

President Bush, Steiger had no medical or public health background when he was appointed director of the government's Office of Global Health Affairs. (He still occupies this post while he awaits Senate confirmation as ambassador to Mozambique.) It is common practice for presidents to appoint well-connected but inexperienced allies to key policy posts. Although they can be depended on to follow the president's political agenda, they often have little or no substantive knowledge about the agencies they administer.

Steiger maintained that the global health report should focus mainly on the steps that the Bush administration had taken to improve health worldwide. Carmona wanted to release a version drafted by international health experts that reviewed the links between poverty and ill health and advocated that disease prevention and treatment become a part of the US's foreign policy. When Steiger wouldn't approve this report, which he called "often inaccurate and out of date," and Carmona refused to release the administration's version, the report was cancelled.

The Bush administration seems more likely than most to suppress scientific information to further political ideology, with recent complaints surfacing from disgruntled employees at the National Institutes of Health, the Food and Drug Administration, and NASA. Such meddling happens in all administrations, though, and it raises two issues that transcend administration and subject matter: what happens when an official disagrees with an announced policy, and what to do when scientific expertise is disregarded and evidence is manipulated or ignored.

In the first of these, the traditional advice to political appointees has been to advocate for their opinions strongly in private discussions but support whatever policy eventually emerges. A well-known example of this was when President Clinton's Health and Human Services Secretary, Donna Shalala, strongly disagreed with making a major change in welfare payment policy that would result in many people being thrown off the welfare lists. But when the president endorsed it she went along publicly, despite opposition from her liberal constituency. Most now agree that it was, on balance, an important and successful reform.

The second issue is trickier. Carmona complained that political ideology was trumping science when, for instance, he was not allowed to advocate any type of sex education for young people except abstinence, even though scientific reviews showed clearly that abstinence-only sex education does not work well. It was reminiscent of an episode in the Reagan administration when then Surgeon General Koop was ordered to prepare a report on the adverse psychological effects of abortion. After reviewing the literature, Koop refused, saying that he had found none. As a conservative surgeon whose appointment was opposed by liberals, he had enough stature and support to weather that particular storm.

Clearly a presidential administration should be allowed to attempt to set its agenda, to focus on what it thinks are important issues, and to prioritize. It also, of course, has a right to tout its accomplishments and take credit for even the serendipitous achievements that have taken place during its tenure. When, however, administration officials knowingly cite inaccurate or misleading information or bend the rules of science or evidence in pursuit of a political agenda or policy, it is a different matter entirely. That is the time for honorable government employees whether career status or political appointees—who are unable to convince the administration to desist from such distortions to call attention to them in the only way they can: resignation.

BMJ, February 9, 2008

What the candidates fail to mention

Primary care is nowhere to be seen, either as a problem or a solution

Although the Iraq war and, more recently, the sad state of the economy have dominated the political campaign for US president, health care problems have continued to be cited by voters as a big concern. Each candidate has a retinue of health care advisers, and their websites are full of position papers and multi-point plans on this topic.

Everyone agrees about the nature of the problem. Health care now consumes 16 percent of the US gross domestic product, and costs continue to climb. We spent about $7,000 per person on health care in 2006, over $2 trillion in all. Around 45 million Americans have no health insurance for at least part of the year. The population is aging. We baby boomers, who expect and consume lots of health care, are now beginning to turn 65. We are going to be a big problem.

But despite all of the money we spend on high-tech medicine, the US is consistently near the bottom of rankings of health care outcomes in developed countries. There are continuing concerns about the quality of health care and medical errors. While most patients like their doctors, they are grossly dissatisfied with the US health care system.

The candidates also more or less agree on many changes that are needed to fix things: an increased focus on preventive medicine, wider use of computerized medical records to decrease errors and improve care, more information for patients, and improved care and coordination for people with chronic diseases.

The candidates differ, though, on the organizing principles behind their prescriptions for change. The Republicans tend to focus on cutting costs and increasing patient choice and control over their health care, usually through some type of market-based solution where people can choose their own privately sponsored insurance. Democrats are for cutting costs too, but they give more attention in their plans to providing insurance coverage for everyone (or almost everyone) as a way to improve health and health care.

Unless I am missing something, however, *all* of the major candidates omit a major issue from their discussions and proposals. My web search of the health care platforms of the candidates failed to find a single mention of the term "primary care." Does no one realize that the current woeful state of primary care medicine in the US is both a likely cause of many of our problems as well a potential solution for them?

The advantages of a strong primary care infrastructure have been well documented in studies around the world. Where there is good primary care, patients have reduced mortality and better outcomes from cardiovascular and pulmonary diseases. They are hospitalized less frequently and use emergency services more appropriately. Strong primary care systems are associated with better delivery of preventive services and better detection of breast, cervical, and colorectal cancers. Patient satisfaction is better in primary care patients. Medical care delivered by primary care clinicians is less costly, with less testing and comparable outcomes. In areas of income inequality, increased primary care services are associated with reduced health disparities.

All of which argues that the US should have a vigorous primary care system. But in fact, primary care in the US is in crisis, and things are getting worse. Currently, primary care doctors, which in the US include general internists and general pediatricians as well as family physicians, comprise about 35 percent of the US medical workforce, compared to 50 percent or more in most industrialized countries. The number of US medical students choosing family medicine residencies decreased by half in the past 10 years, as did the proportion of internal medicine residents who planned careers in primary care instead of a subspecialty. So not only are there too few American primary care doctors, but their numbers are likely to decrease in the foreseeable future.

This is not surprising, given that the median income of primary care doctors in the US is only slightly more than half of that of subspecialists. Graduating internists who go into primary care can expect to earn at most half of what their medical subspecialty colleagues make. Primary care doctors see more patients than subspecialists, and yet their income, adjusted for inflation, declined by 10 percent from 1995 to 2002.

What will it take to reverse these trends? What can the presidential candidates propose that would make a difference? Much of the needed reform is financial. Primary care doctors should be paid more. Care that is continuous and coordinated should be rewarded. Health-related counseling and other time-intensive but low-tech services should be reimbursed generously.

Subsidies could be used to increase student incentives to enter primary care training programs. Similar incentives could be provided to medical schools and hospitals to partially offset trainee salaries. Loan forgiveness programs for primary care doctors would make higher paying subspecialties less attractive and ease young doctors' transition into primary care practice. Finally, the practice of primary care medicine should be improved by providing increased support for preventive care, better reimbursement for nontraditional service provision (such as group and e-mail care), and more incentives for health care delivery by primary care teams.

Primary care medicine is a crucial missing piece of the health care puzzle. It needs to be a part of the proposals of all the presidential candidates.

BMJ, October 18, 2008

A cautionary tale for the presidential candidates

A look back at the Bush administration's record on health

With the US economy in shambles, it is hard for the presidential candidates to talk about anything else. The small amount of newsprint and bandwidth available for other issues is devoted to Iraq, Afghanistan, and terrorism. Nobody is focusing much on health care and science policy any more. When health care is discussed, it is mainly about coverage and cost: how can we change our health care "system" to take care of more of our population and afford to pay for it? Pundits proclaim that health care reform will be unachievable in the next president's first term because there is no money to do it and no energy for anything but the economy and the war. This is depressing.

One thing that doesn't depend on funding, however, could be done immediately by the next president: reverse the unprecedented policies of George W. Bush's administration that have subverted scientific integrity throughout the government.

The Union of Concerned Scientists has documented dozens of examples over the past eight years of direct interference with government scientists and their work in the service of the administration's political beliefs and goals. The examples range across the scientific agencies of the government and cover topics from the environment to pollution and contamination to national security. Examples from public health include

- Insisting on and publicizing the effectiveness of abstinence-only sex education, despite a lack of evidence for it,

- Censoring testimony before Congress by the Centers for Disease Control and Prevention (CDC) on the health hazards of climate change,

- Posting erroneous data linking abortions and breast cancer on CDC's website,

- Distorting evidence on the effectiveness of condoms in preventing HIV transmission and prevention,

- "Stacking" a federal advisory committee on prevention of lead poisoning to prevent more stringent standards, and

- Adding non-scientific proponents of positions favored by the administration to sessions at scientific meetings, in the guise of providing "balance."

Every incoming president has a political agenda that he wants to promote throughout the government, the nation, and the world. For example, it was no secret that Bush was against abortion. When he took office in 2001, he immediately ended support for all foreign aid to family planning clinics that counseled patients on abortion as an option, even if the funds for abortions were not supplied by the US aid. One can argue (and I believe) that this was a harmful action that should not have been done, but it was at least presented honestly as a policy decision, not a scientific one. People who were against it could lobby for its reversal, and those who voted for Bush could see clearly that this was a direct result of their vote for his anti-abortion views.

Similarly, all administrations want to present their accomplishments in the best possible light. So it is not surprising that they would prefer that all their policy interventions work, that all health trends be positive, and that good news be the only kind of news that emerges. It is also expected that they will try to put the best possible "spin" on results that are not positive. Spin, however, is not the same as distorting science in the service of politics.

A case in point is the delay in approval by the Food and Drug Administration (FDA) of over-the-counter sales of the emergency contraceptive *Plan B*. Despite overwhelming evidence of the drug's safety and effectiveness, the FDA delayed approval for more than 3 years from the time its own advisory committee recommended it by a vote of 23 to 4, officially citing concerns about skimpy data on 14- to 16-year-olds. In fact, the concern was the widely publicized but inaccurate "fact" that *Plan B* worked by preventing implantation and thus caused abortions.

The Bush administration's attack on scientific truth has not been limited to contraception and abortion. It refused to publish scientific evidence of the extent of racial disparities in health outcomes and health care in the United States that were assembled by government scientists for a congressionally mandated report. It repeatedly allowed bogus "science" to be presented by special interest groups to "balance" discussions and to delay and sometimes reverse environmental health decisions supported by valid evidence. It prevented its own surgeon general from speaking out on topics in the areas of mental health, global health, and secondhand smoking. It rigged testing and fudged results of formaldehyde level testing in government-supplied trailer homes for victims of Hurricane Katrina. And it fired or did not reappoint members of dozens of federal advisory committees who did not agree with Bush's views. Friends and former colleagues throughout the government have told me that the extent of falsification and suppression of scientific evidence by this administration is unprecedented.

So what should a President McCain or Obama do about all this? During his first week in office the new president could issue an executive order supporting unimpeded scientific research, the primacy of peer review, and the freedom of government scientists to submit their research results for publication. He could pledge not to interfere with the scientific processes and activities of government agencies. And he could encourage transparency and public scrutiny of appointment procedures of advisory and review committees. This is a low-cost policy change that has a good chance of improving the health of all Americans.

BMJ, January 17, 2009

What should the surgeon general do?

Sanjay Gupta is a television star—but the problem lies elsewhere

As I write this, it is being widely reported that the neurosurgeon Sanjay Gupta, who is also a medical correspondent for CNN and CBS, is the leading candidate to be appointed surgeon general by the president-elect, Barack Obama. I have nothing against Gupta, who I am sure is a fine neurosurgeon, specializing (according to his biography) in "complicated spine, trauma and 3-D image-guided operations." He is also a skilled television medical correspondent. His potential appointment, however, raises two important issues about the role of what everyone calls the "surgeon general of the United States."

The first is that the surgeon general is actually statutorily only the surgeon general of the Commissioned Corps of the US Public Health Service. The corps comprises more than 6,000 uniformed officers who work in public health positions throughout the federal government and on assignment in public health agencies around the nation and the world. It is not clear what qualifies a neurosurgeon with no public health background to lead this uniformed service.

Second, and more importantly, I am concerned at reports that Gupta has been offered a major role in the White House Office of Health Reform, working with the Health and Human Services secretary-designate, Tom Daschle, to create and pass health care reform legislation. If this is true, it reflects a fundamental misunderstanding by the Obama administration of the role—and potential contributions—of the surgeon general.

We certainly need health care reform in the US, and it is good news that the Obama administration is going to make it a priority issue. It will be, however, a contentious, highly political struggle. If Gupta, with his background in the Clinton administration and his communication skills, wants to work on changing the US health care system, that's great. The president should appoint him to the White House staff or make him the assistant secretary for health and let him go at it. But not surgeon general.

The most important traditional role for the surgeon general, the one that the nation knows about, is not the statutory one. It is to provide impartial, independent, evidence-based advice to the president and the country about health and disease. This is the reason that everyone thinks of him or her as the "nation's chief doctor." If the surgeon general is seen as just another adviser to the president or as an administration spokesperson on health, the result is a huge loss of credibility and effectiveness.

There are many recent examples of surgeons general successfully taking on this role. The most notable was Luther Terry, who issued a landmark report in 1964 that unequivocally linked smoking and cancer. This came at a time when almost half of American adults smoked. Terry later recalled that he chose a Saturday for the press release of his report, to minimize the effect on the stock market and to maximize coverage in the Sunday papers. The report "hit the country like a bombshell" and was "front page news and a lead story on every radio and television station in the United States and many abroad."

Another example was C. Everett Koop's courageous insistence in 1986 on reporting the facts about how HIV infection is spread. Despite concerns from both conservatives in the Reagan administration and gay rights activists on the left, Koop graphically described what was known about risky sexual behavior to all Americans. He sent a mailing on AIDS to every household in the country.

And, in 1999, Surgeon General David Satcher issued an important report on mental illness in America that documented the disparities in health care and coverage for people with mental disorders. Only last year were these issues finally addressed, with congressional passage of the Mental Health Parity Act of 2008, mandating equal insurance coverage for treatment of mental disorders.

These and other crucial public health achievements could never have been accomplished if the surgeon general had been just another member of the president's political team, trying to get his programs passed. This is why the surgeon general's appointment is for a fixed term of 4 years, which does not necessarily coincide with the term of the president and his other appointees. The surgeon general must be independent and not identified with any of the president's personal agenda. The easiest way to do this would be for Obama to appoint a current senior career officer in the Public Health

Service to be surgeon general, just as career officers are appointed to be the surgeons general of the US Army, Navy, and Air Force.

The argument for Gupta's appointment is, of course, that he already has a national following that would allow him to stand up to political attempts to silence him. But if the Obama administration does wish to appoint Gupta, it should first decide whether it wants him to be their front man for health care reform—which I'm sure he could do very capably—or whether it wants him to do something else entirely: to be the surgeon general of the United States.

BMJ, February 14, 2009

The taxing case of Tom Daschle

A lesson for the new president, perhaps with wide ranging consequences

The former US senator Tom Daschle seemed like the perfect candidate to lead President Obama's effort for health care reform and to serve as his Health and Human Services secretary. As a former Senate majority leader, Daschle knew both the players and the processes necessary to get legislation through Congress. He coauthored a book on health care reform and was passionately interested in the topic. As one of Obama's earliest supporters and advisers, he was likely to have the president's confidence and attention. Daschle had led the Obama health transition team since the election; conducted numerous discussion sessions with citizens and experts on health care reform during the interregnum; and was awaiting Senate confirmation.

Yet, in a stunning reversal of fortune, this consummate insider felt it necessary to withdraw his name from consideration just days before he was likely to be confirmed by the Senate and sworn in. What happened and what does it mean for the president's agenda in general and health care reform in particular?

After being defeated by the Republicans for re-election in 2004, Daschle left the Senate but not Washington. Though not a lawyer, he joined the law and lobbying firm Alston and Bird and provided advice to clients about how to deal with Congress. His advice and connections were apparently enough to earn him a seven-figure salary. He also traveled the country, giving speeches to dozens of organizations that were happy to pay him $10,000 or more to hear his opinions on policy matters. In addition, Daschle advised an investment fund, which also paid him well and provided him with a car and driver. A standard career after federal service for senior legislators who, like the missionaries in Hawaii, came to do good and did well.

It is a bit unfair to paint the former senator as a money hungry sell-out, though. He also served as an unpaid fellow at the Center for American Progress, a liberal think tank, where he collaborated with staff there on his health care reform book. He was a visiting fellow at Georgetown University's

Public Policy Institute, where he conducted a popular series of policy seminars with visiting Washington luminaries. Plus, he was careful not to actually lobby his former Senate colleagues by going back to Capitol Hill and importuning them on behalf of his clients.

All was going swimmingly until it was announced that Daschle had not paid taxes on the value of the car and driver that had been supplied to him and thus owed over $100,000 in back taxes, penalties, and interest. He paid up just before he was to appear before various Senate committees for questioning. In the context of similar tax delinquencies uncovered in two other senior Obama appointees, this led to strong criticism from the press, Republicans, and some Democrats. It seemed contradictory both to the ethical positions that Obama had campaigned on and the restrictions against hiring former lobbyists he had imposed on himself. Indeed, many felt that the published list of health-related organizations that had paid hundreds of thousands of dollars to hear Daschle speak was more damaging to his candidacy than the unpaid taxes. In response to the criticism, and despite still being likely to be confirmed, Daschle withdrew his name from consideration, some say only a step ahead of a request from Obama to do so.

Then, in a truly remarkable reaction to this problem, Obama took the offensive and used five different previously scheduled prime-time television interviews to apologize and take responsibility for the mistake of appointing Daschle. "I screwed up," he said, in a shocking admission for any president to make. You cannot imagine either of his two predecessors voluntarily owning up to an error of this sort.

Which leads to the most important question about all of this: What will be the fallout? Narrowly, most commentators feel that Daschle will be hard to replace as the leader of Obama's health reform effort. His combination of policy knowledge and political skill was close to unique. It will likely delay the initiative by weeks if not months, and it may threaten it altogether.

There may also be broader implications, in two areas. First, the Daschle debacle may affect the selection process for future senior appointees, both assuring that they are not tax delinquents but more importantly by shining a light on their former financial dealings with the industries they will be regulating. It would be more than a small victory if in the future the Washington revolving door didn't spin quite so quickly or effortlessly.

Second, it is interesting to speculate about the effect of this episode on the very young presidency of Barack Obama. To the extent it delays or prevents health care reform, its effect is negative. To the extent that admitting a mistake casts the president as inexperienced and incompetent, its effect is very negative. Another way to look at it, however, is that it is rather refreshing and even admirable to see a president struggling to act consistently with his professed ideals and admitting when he comes up short.

BMJ, March 28, 2009

The papal position on condoms and HIV

It would be a blessing if Benedict XVI could stop advocating policies that endanger health

When I was 6 years old or so I used to go through my father's top dresser drawer looking for pennies. One day I found a strange rubber balloon wrapped in foil. I didn't know what it was and didn't recognize the big word printed on the outside of the wrapper: "prophylactic" (this was the genteel 1950s). An inquisitive child, I looked it up in the dictionary and found out that the word meant "acting to defend or prevent something, especially a disease." I idly wondered what disease my father was trying to prevent with this balloon but soon lost interest.

I thought of this memory when I read about Pope Benedict XVI's recent comments about the use of condoms to prevent HIV transmission. As I write this, news accounts of his recent trip to Africa have been dominated by reactions to comments he made as he was flying there from Rome. He was quoted as saying that AIDS "can't be resolved with the distribution of condoms." "On the contrary," he said, "it increases the problem." Health officials and editorialists around the world have strongly objected to the pope's statement, but I think that there is more to the story than just correcting his facts.

It is no surprise, of course, that the pope is against the use of condoms and supports sexual abstinence as the best way to prevent the spread of HIV. He rejects condom use as part of the Catholic Church's position against what it terms "artificial contraception." As many have already pointed out, however, the pope was just plain wrong when he said that condoms make the AIDS problem worse.

Many studies done around the world, including in Africa, have found that condom use can decrease the risk of HIV transmission by about 80 percent—not perfect, by any means, but an effective strategy. For instance, analyses have shown that the famous "ABC" (abstain, be faithful, condom use) program in Uganda, which was successful in decreasing the number of new cases of AIDS, probably owed most of its effectiveness to greater use of condoms.

A second concern is the pope's position that fidelity within and abstinence outside marriage obviates the need for condoms to prevent the spread of HIV. While such behavior—though difficult to attain—would certainly help, this position ignores the reality of family life in sub-Saharan Africa. There, much of the spread of HIV occurs within, not outside, marriages, from infected husbands having unprotected sex with their wives. If condoms are not available, these women are forced to make the impossible choice between refusing to have sex with their husbands (and risking abuse) or consenting to sex (and risking HIV infection).

Some argue that critics of the Catholic Church's position on condom use are wrong when they say that it will be likely to lead to a greater spread of HIV. They say that anyone observant enough to follow the church's teachings on condoms will also adhere to its policies on sexual abstinence before and fidelity within marriage. I'm not sure where the evidence for this position comes from; I can't imagine that many Catholics are any different from many Jews or Muslims in selective observance of commandments. Furthermore, this position completely ignores the pope's influence on non-Catholic Christians and others.

Others state that if Catholic rules about condom use were an independent risk factor, then African countries with a higher proportion of Catholics would have higher HIV infection rates, which they don't. We know, however, that correlations, or the lack of correlations, cannot be accepted as arguments for or against causality. In addition, this view certainly discounts the hugely important effect of the many wonderful Catholic missionaries who provide health care and social services throughout Africa and the developing world, regardless of the local religions, and who cannot advocate condom use.

One possible approach to the seemingly irresolvable conflict between condoms and religious dictums might be to separate the disease prevention attributes of condoms from their contraceptive effect. There is precedent for this, at least in the United States. Many Catholic hospitals and doctors here prescribe oral contraceptives to women not to prevent pregnancy but instead to prevent heavy, painful periods. Would it be too much of a stretch to imagine the Catholic Church tacitly condoning condom use as part of an overall disease prevention program to decrease the spread of HIV, even if only within marriages?

That is where my childhood memory kicks in. We could advocate using prophylactics in the dictionary sense of the word I learned when I was 6—preventing disease instead of babies.

The pope's job is to be the spiritual leader of the world's Catholics. It would be a true blessing if he could do that without advocating policies that endanger the health of some of the world's neediest people.

BMJ, July 17, 2010

The case of the sugar-sweetened beverage tax

A cautionary tale of political influence

We are fat, and we're getting fatter. Nearly a third of American children are overweight or obese. In our inner cities a prevalence of obesity of more than 50 percent among both children and adults is not uncommon. Too many calories in, too little energy out.

Changing behavior is hard. Obesity has several causes, and it will take a multifaceted campaign to reverse the trend. The tobacco experience has taught us that education is not enough; regulation, litigation, and legislation are needed, too. Increasing taxes on cigarettes has been the single most effective strategy in reducing smoking.

Which brings us to the sad story of the tax on sugar sweetened beverages (SSBs).

An important part of the obesity story is clearly the huge increase in consumption of SSBs: carbonated sodas, sweet teas, energy drinks, flavored water, and sports drinks. Their use has more than doubled in recent years, and of all food types they are the single largest contributor to energy intake in the United States.

Especially perniciously, SSBs have essentially no effect on satiety, research shows, unlike candy or other junk food. Our bodies seem not to sense the empty calories we're swallowing and to count them toward feeling full. Gobble some jelly beans and you feel like you've had something to eat. Drink a cola drink—no such feeling. Add in the fact that the price of SSBs has actually fallen after adjustment for inflation and you have the makings of a big problem.

Experts have been agitating for a "penny per ounce" tax on SSBs for about 2 years. An excise tax imposed at the wholesale level has several advantages over a percentage sales tax collected at the cash register after the purchases have been totaled. Because it is imposed at the wholesale level, an excise tax is easier to implement. It is then passed on to the consumer in higher retail prices, allowing price sensitivity to work its magic. Also, it produces the same tax on a discounted generic soda as on a brand name drink. Thus, rather than driving people to purchase cheaper products or larger serving sizes to get a better price, as a sales tax does, excise taxes can actually reduce consumption. What amounts to about a 10 percent tax will likely lead to an 8–10 percent reduction in consumption.

Just as with tobacco products, we especially want to discourage young people from buying and consuming SSBs, and the young are notoriously price-sensitive. Poor people, who are disproportionately obese, are the most price sensitive of all in food shopping.

Simple sales taxes have been shown not to work. They don't change behavior or weight. The best chance for success is to impose a penny per ounce SSB tax, resulting in a rise of a dollar or two in the price of a six-pack of sodas or a 2 liter bottle. Pilot studies and some early research have found promising decreases in consumption and even positive health outcomes from such pricing strategies. Public opinion polls have found that most people are in favor of such taxes. It seems like a pretty good public health strategy.

Needless to say, SSB manufacturers and retailers did not think these taxes were a very good idea at all. This was a threat they would beat back at any cost.

The industry's response to proposed SSB taxes has been swift and massive. In cities and states where SSB taxes have been proposed, industry-financed "grassroots" organizations sprang up out of nowhere. They had names like "New Yorkers Against Unfair Taxes" and "NoDCBevTax.com." Their websites listed dozens of ordinary citizens and small mom-and-pop stores as members, masking the source of their funding: the major soft drink companies and retailers.

In New York State, projections found that a penny per ounce tax on SSBs could prevent 145,000 cases of adult obesity and 37,000 cases of diabetes in a decade. It could save $2 billion in health care costs. To fight the tax, SSB manufacturers paid $90 million to the same public relations firm that created the famed "Harry and Louise" advertisements against US health reform in the 1990s. Their signature New York TV spot showed a housewife urging viewers to "tell Albany to trim their budget fat and leave our groceries alone." The governor withdrew his tax proposal.

Washington, DC, was another battleground: a liberal, black-majority city with chronically underperforming schools and a large budget deficit.

A city council member proposed a penny per ounce SSB tax to decrease obesity and fund better school food and exercise programs. Immediately, we heard insulting but effective radio advertisements with stereotyped African American voices saying that "soda's 'bout to git waaay more expensive" because of unfair taxes. It wasn't even a close contest. The city council chairman never called for a vote on the proposal.

The story was the same around the US. In many cities and states, proposals were withdrawn in the face of "public" protest and petitions. In others, excise taxes were converted to ineffective sales taxes. Public health was outgunned and outspent. SSBs are still safe for all to buy and enjoy at record low prices.

As the mayor of Philadelphia said about the victory of the beverage lobby's campaign, "They're successful the old-fashioned way. They pay for it."

BMJ, August 28, 2010

Smoking or obesity: must we target only one?

Funds for anti-obesity campaigns increase while tobacco programs languish

In a landmark article published almost 20 years ago, McGinnis and Foege showed that the actual leading causes of death in the United States were not cardiovascular disease and cancer, which had long led the "leading causes" rankings calculated from death certificate analyses. Using data cobbled together from a number of sources, they estimated that smoking, with 400,000 deaths a year, and diseases related to diet and lack of physical activity, with 300,000 deaths, were in fact the leading killers of Americans. Together they caused about a third of all deaths in 1990.

The headlines then were all about how smoking was at the top of the list and that almost half of that year's deaths were a result of it and other preventable, behavior-related causes. Many people were also surprised at the huge toll taken by poor diet and lack of physical activity, but it wasn't a focus of discussion.

The intervening decades have been a terrific success story for anti-tobacco efforts. As a result of an effective, multi-tiered campaign, including higher taxes on tobacco, bans on smoking indoors, targeted counter-marketing, cessation help lines, drugs, and counseling, the prevalence of smoking in the has fallen to around 20 percent in American adults—less than half what it was in 1955.

The past few years have seen increasing attention on another public health problem: obesity. It has threatened to dethrone tobacco as the number one public health catastrophe in the making. Indeed, a redo of the McGinnis and Foege analysis 10 years later found that, while tobacco was still in the lead in 2000, with 435,000 attributed deaths, diet and activity (largely obesity-related) deaths had risen to 365,000 a year. The authors cautioned that "poor diet and physical inactivity may soon overtake tobacco as the leading cause of death."

Obesity is a huge problem that is probably getting worse. The prevalence of childhood obesity has tripled among school-age children and adolescents since 1980, and more than 70 million US adults are now obese. Obese adults and children have an increased risk of several chronic diseases and incur dramatically increased health care costs.

The anti-tobacco strategies were not lost on those trying to combat obesity. The same multi-focal approach that worked so well for smokers is being applied to obesity. Interventions currently under way range from regulatory to legislative to clinical. In fact, public health attention and funding have now tilted toward obesity. A recent iconic photo of the first lady, Michelle Obama, says it all. She was shown on the south lawn of the White House vigorously exercising with a group of kids at the kick-off of her anti-obesity "Let's move!" campaign. Needless to say, no similar anti-tobacco campaign is being led by her reportedly still-smoking husband.

A recent article in the *New York Times* described how public health funding, from both government and private sources, has shifted from tobacco to obesity in the US. The country's largest health charity, the Robert Wood Johnson Foundation, which funded many of the tobacco policy initiatives that have been so successful, has now decreased its anti-tobacco funding in favor of a $500 million anti-obesity campaign. Federal stimulus money earmarked for prevention has funded both tobacco and obesity efforts, but recently obesity programs have received more than tobacco. States have had to cut their budgets and have decreased spending on tobacco. All of this has preventionistas like me worried. How do we decide whether to fund anti-tobacco or anti-obesity campaigns?

On the one hand, while tobacco control programs have been a poster child for success, the war is not over. The downward trend in smoking seems to have stalled; prevalence has hovered around 20 percent since 2006. Some 450,000 Americans still die each year from tobacco-related illness, and more than 8 million are sick or disabled because of it. Further, smoking and smoking-related diseases are now more than ever a class phenomenon. More vulnerable people smoke, including poor people, many ethnic minority groups, and people with chronic mental illnesses. Don't forget that the tobacco companies are still out there pitching, trying to recruit new smokers to replace those who die or quit.

On the other hand, at least trends in smoking have long been going in the right direction. The obesity problem seems to be getting worse. Also, anti-tobacco efforts have a new champion now that the Food and Drug

Administration has regulatory authority over tobacco and a new office and staff to make and enforce its rules.

One big test for federal funding will come as the new Affordable Care Act (health care reform) goes into effect. One provision of the law calls for increasingly large amounts of public funding for public health and prevention, starting with $500 million in 2010 and rising to $1 billion a year by 2012. How much of this investment, totaling $15 billion, will go to anti-obesity efforts and how much to tobacco?

The lobbyists are lining up, but in this case they are all lobbyists for the "good guys." Maybe there will be enough money to go around for both worthy causes. Funding to combat the two leading causes of death in America—whatever their rank order—should not have to be a zero-sum game.

BMJ, January 29, 2011

Guns don't kill crowds, people with semiautomatics do

Why can't we do a better job of protecting society from this type of attack?

Once again in the United States, a seriously mentally ill man is suspected of mowing down a crowd before he can be wrestled to the ground.

This time the victims included a congresswoman and a federal judge. A wave of shock spread across the country and around the world. Liberals blamed the mood of the country and violent rhetoric from conservative leaders. Conservatives howled with injustice and attacked the liberals for attacking them.

The handgun used for the attack was a Glock 19, a lightweight, compact, semiautomatic pistol that comes with a standard magazine holding 15 bullets of 9 mm caliber. Glock pistols have become the overwhelming choice of police departments around the world because of their light polymer construction and their ease of firing. They are called "semiautomatic" guns because, unlike revolvers that have one bullet per chamber, all the bullets can be fired by simply squeezing and re-squeezing the trigger. Jared Loughner, the alleged gunman, had legally purchased this weapon in November, along with an extended capacity magazine that allowed him to fire 33 times without stopping to reload.

Loughner, 22, was clearly mentally ill. Press reports after the event have documented a mind unraveling and descending into madness over the previous year. He lost his friends. He had repeated run-ins with school authorities. He disrupted his college classes, and classmates sat next to the door, fearing that he might get violent. He posted bizarre theories and claims on Internet sites, leading one regular poster to label him as having schizophrenia and to plead with him to get help or start taking his medications again. He had several encounters with the police, including one on the day of the shooting. But no one made a formal complaint, and Loughner never received a psychiatric evaluation.

Ever responsive, the US Congress immediately sprang into action to fix the problem. One congressman introduced legislation making it a crime to carry a gun within 1,000 feet of a member of Congress. Laughably unenforceable, patently self-protectionist, and just plain silly, it seemed the perfect response to the tragedy. In fact, no legislation is likely to be passed in response to this event.

The second amendment to the US Constitution states that "the right of the people to keep and bear arms shall not be infringed." Americans, with the exception of some pockets of opposition on the two coasts, believe that citizens have a right to own and carry guns. Apparently most of us like having guns around, and there is no chance that any laws will be passed to limit access to them significantly. No amount of handgun-related violence and no high-profile killings will change this.

Three years ago a similarly deranged young man, Seung-Hui Cho, killed 32 fellow students at a Virginia university. He used a Glock 19 as well. His rampage did lead to changes in state and national laws to make it more difficult for mentally ill people to buy guns. Unfortunately such restrictions work only if a person is in the mental health system, and Loughner never made it that far.

We are told that guns don't kill people, that people kill people, and that what we have here is a failure of the mental health treatment system, not the legal system. But in order to kill a lot of people fast before being stopped, even crazy people need access to guns that are easy to fire and have lots of bullets in them.

I don't think the problem is the mood of the country or who was placed in Sarah Palin's cross-hairs in her campaign literature. There will always be seriously disturbed individuals out there who, because of our country's history and experience, will have a chance to access guns. Given that we have no realistic chance of banning handguns, if we have any hope of preventing such future tragedies there are only two things we can do.

First, we need to prevent the sale of equipment that facilitates such easy carnage: high-capacity magazines for easily concealed guns. What is the purpose of a 33-shot magazine for a Glock? Who needs to fire 33 times without reloading? If Loughner had had a revolver instead of a 33-shot Glock he would have succeeded in shooting his target but probably not many more people. Cho would have had to stop to reload more often and likely could have been stopped short of killing 32 others.

Second, it must be made clear that it is everyone's job to report obviously disturbed people and get them into treatment. Neither Loughner nor Cho was a close call. Many people sensed that they were dangers to themselves and others. If someone had stepped up and reported Loughner, he might have had a paper trail that would have prevented him from buying his gun.

Guns don't kill crowds, but mentally disturbed people with high capacity semiautomatic pistols do.

BMJ, March 19, 2011

The rise and likely fall of Don Berwick

What can be learned from this appointment disappointment at Medicare?

Democrats have given up hope of saving Donald Berwick, the current director of the influential and costly US Medicare and Medicaid health insurance programs. He will now likely lose his job at the end of the year. It is a disturbing and discouraging development, worth reviewing for possible lessons learned.

The Centers for Medicare & Medicaid Services (officially abbreviated, incorrectly, as CMS) is the proverbial 800 pound gorilla of US health care. Its Medicare program pays for care for most Americans aged 65 and older, and its state-based Medicaid program covers uninsured poor people. More than 100 million Americans have CMS-administered insurance. The administration asked Congress for just under $850 *billion* to fund CMS next year, and its programs are growing as Americans age and more of the poor are covered under health reform's Affordable Care Act.

In addition to its direct role in paying hospitals and doctors for care, CMS has a huge influence on private-sector insurance as well. Because of its size, CMS sets standards for coverage policies and payment levels that are almost universally adopted (or at least adapted) by private health plans and insurance companies. So the head of CMS—in government-speak, the administrator—is a key position indeed.

Soon after his election in 2008, President Obama made many key health sector appointments, but he chose not to appoint a CMS administrator. Once health reform passed last March it became even more vital to have someone running CMS. Finally, a month later, Obama nominated Berwick to be CMS administrator.

It is hard to imagine a more inspiring, exciting, and forward-looking nominee than Don Berwick, a pediatrician who has spent much of his career focusing on improving the quality and safety of health care. His experience in improving quality and safety in hospitals and medical practices would seem to be exactly what the huge federal systems needed, not to mention his charismatic leadership style. I first met and worked with Don in the early 1990s, when he was vice-chair of the US Preventive Services Task Force. It was clear then that he was a brilliant thinker and a dynamic, even inspirational, leader. He went on to found and lead the Institute for Healthcare Improvement, a private, not-for-profit organization that works with hospitals, health systems, and practices to find measurable ways to improve quality and safety and cut waste and needless expense. He also co-authored two hugely influential reports from the US Institute of Medicine, *To Err is Human* and *Crossing the Quality Chasm*.

Senate confirmation is required for appointments at this level, but the necessary hearings for Berwick were never scheduled. The administration blamed Congress, saying that they had delayed considering the appointment for political reasons. Not at all, responded Congress, blaming the administration and Berwick for dragging their feet in providing necessary background information. The nomination went nowhere.

In July, tired of waiting, the president bypassed the Senate's confirmation powers by using a mechanism called a "recess appointment" to install Berwick as CMS administrator unilaterally. This loophole, roundly condemned and yet widely used by all presidents, was designed to keep the government running during long periods in which the Congress was not in session. Obama appointed Berwick during the week-long July 4th break, hardly meeting the intent of a recess appointment.

Republicans were incensed, and even many Democrats were disappointed that they did not have a chance to question Berwick before he took office. It is easy to find quotes from his long career that upset conservative free-market Republicans, including discussions of how the US already rations health care and praise for the many accomplishments of the United Kingdom's National Health Service.

Recess appointments expire with the end of a 2-year congressional session, in this case December 2011. Presumably the administration hoped that Berwick could mend fences with enough Republicans to allow him to be renominated and (this time) properly confirmed by the Senate before then. It hasn't happened. On March 1, 42 Republican Senators wrote Obama to urge him to withdraw Berwick's renomination because of the way he was appointed the first time, the now-expanded role of CMS under health reform, and his "lack of experience" and prior "controversial statements."

How could this have happened? A visionary nominee, thought by many to be one of Obama's best appointments, who was endorsed by medical organizations, public health leaders, hospitals, and virtually everyone else in organized health care, is going to be scuttled after 18 months in office.

Perhaps it could not have been avoided, as the poisonous atmosphere between Republicans and Democrats seems to intrude at every level, especially where health care reform is concerned and given the many new "Tea Party" members of Congress. Maybe, however, the president should not have waited until reform had passed to name his CMS leader, and maybe he should not have used the recess appointment to install him without hearings. It might have taken longer to get him into office, but perhaps Berwick would have ended up with more time—more than the 18 months he will likely have—to make the changes he needs and wants to make in the US health care system.

As the *Washington Post* pundit Ezra Klein said, both Berwick and the Medicare and Medicaid recipients he could have helped deserved better than this.

4

Health Care Reform

"Health is a blessing that money cannot buy."
—Isaac Walton, 1593–1683

For Americans involved in health care, the central issue of our time is our expensive, high-tech, infuriating health care system. As we approach spending 20 percent of our annual gross domestic product on health care, we somehow continue to exclude almost that percentage of residents from decent insurance coverage. Surveys show that we like our doctors but not anything else about our system.

After the election of 2008, it looked like the timing was perfect for change. Increasing costs and dissatisfaction with health care and a seemingly bullet-proof Democratic majority in Congress led many to think that the newly elected president could succeed where others had failed. Reform of health care delivery and coverage was just a matter of time and presidential leadership, we thought.

As it turned out, of course, the bullet-proof congressional majority was lost in an upset in a special election for a Massachusetts Senate seat. The road to a new health care system was full of ups and downs and alternating hope and despair. Almost everyone was dissatisfied with the result, signed into law in March of 2010. Since then, the struggle has continued, some trying to explain the new law and begin its implementation while others work to curtail its reach and repeal it.

This section of the book contains essays written while what Democrats call the "Affordable Care Act" and Republicans call "Obamacare" was created, debated, and passed. The commentaries cover many of the major questions that were being discussed: mandating coverage, managing costs, debating comprehensiveness, including preventive medicine, and increasing primary care. I have not re-edited columns in which my predictions turned out to be completely wrong, as I think they accurately represent the feelings of many at the time.

Two of the pieces focus on comparative effectiveness research (CER), which is intended to provide patients, policy makers, and clinicians with information about which drugs and procedures work for which patients. CER was portrayed by participants in the health care reform drama as either a panacea or the devil's work. The truth, of course, is that it is neither. The controversy around it is, however, emblematic of the mix of serious debate and political posturing that has characterized much of this tumultuous period.

BMJ, November 29, 2008

Our perfectly designed health care system

An interregnum thought experiment

The interregnum between a presidential election and the inauguration is a time of feverish activity, in which the president-elect and his staff decide who will help them govern and what they will try to do first. The press and pundits speculate breathlessly on who will be appointed and what they will do first. As I write this, for example, we have just learned that the new administration's secretary of Health and Human Services is likely to be a respected former US senator, Tom Daschle.* He has written a book about health care reform, which is likely to be his assignment when he starts in January.

I've been musing about the United States and how perfectly designed our current health care system is. Perfectly designed, of course, as every system is, to achieve exactly the results it gets, as quality improvement guru Don Berwick has famously said. In its own way, our system is really rather remarkable. Here's a thought experiment to illustrate what I mean.

Suppose you have a big industrialized country that has lots of money to devote to health care: around $2 trillion a year. That is $6,400 per person, far more than any other country spends on health care. Let's say, for the sake of the argument, that the country leads the world in technological advances, developing everything from computers to new scanners before anyone else. We'll also give you a large and enormously profitable drug industry to develop and test new products. Throw in some of the world's best health and health care researchers, well funded by the world's richest health research institutes and foundations. To make sure that all this largesse is fairly distributed, we'll even make this mythical country a democracy, where the voice of the people rules.

Your assignment, should you choose to accept it, is to take all of these resources and design a scenario (notice that I did not say a system) in which both health care process measures and health outcomes in the population

---

*   This, of course, turned out not to be true; see page 79.

are paradoxically poor by international standards. So, despite the money, the technology, and the research talent, you have to find a way to keep neonatal mortality from falling and life expectancy from rising; a way to deliver suboptimal care for people with chronic diseases; and a way to keep delivery of appropriate preventive services uneven and inconsistent. In general, you have to ensure that you are getting poor value for your health care dollar.

This is not easy to do. Most countries would fail, but in the US we did it. The foundation of the scheme is disparity. First, deny health insurance to 47 million people to delay or prevent access to health care. Add another 16 million who are underinsured, so that a catastrophic health event bankrupts them. Create broad disparities in income, so that some people can't afford to pay for insurance or health care. Make sure to tie most health insurance to employment, so that when people lose their jobs they also risk losing their insurance.

Second, make sure that there are no national systems of care or planning to allocate resources evenly across the population. This will allow every facility that wants a magnetic resonance imaging scanner to get one, even if the city already has dozens of MRIs, and it will lead to a high proportion of unnecessary scans, perhaps 20 percent to 30 percent. While we're at it, let's make sure that electronic health care records are adopted by fewer than 20 percent of doctors. That will ensure that medical records and health information are not transferred with the patient, which makes for many more needless tests and miscommunications. It will also impede improvements in continuity of care and patient safety.

Third, spend lots of money, say $300 billion or so a year, on drugs and devices, and allow drugs to be advertised directly to the consumer to keep demand high for new, expensive ones. The drug industry knows that every dollar spent on advertising to patients yields $4 in increased revenues.

Finally, none of this will work unless we make sure that no one is around to coordinate patients' care, to serve as their medical "home," and to deliver necessary preventive treatment and care for acute and chronic disease from cradle to grave. Most countries in the world entrust this job to primary care doctors, who generally make up about 60 percent of the medical workforce. In 1949, 59 percent of US doctors were general practitioners, so we really had to work hard to eliminate them if we were going to achieve our goals. Again, it wasn't easy, but we did it. We made primary care less prestigious than specialty practice. Our multiple payers ensured that most of doctors' time would be spent on paperwork rather than on care of patients. We paid primary care doctors less, a lot less, than subspecialists. And, in a recent clever touch, we dramatically increased the cost of medical school, so that students graduate with hundreds of thousands of dollars of debt, precluding them from choosing a career in primary care. Bingo. Now we have a situation where only 30 or 35 percent of doctors are generalists, and the number is sinking fast.

So there you have it, Mr. Health Secretary-designate. That's how we did it. Good old American ingenuity. It's a mess, for lots of reasons. But it's our mess. How to fix it? That's your job.

BMJ, June 20, 2009

How to waste a billion dollars

Comparative effectiveness research risks ineffectiveness if industry opposition to it succeeds

Comparative effectiveness research (CER) is all the rage in the United States right now. It seems that everywhere you turn, a conference or meeting or briefing on CER is being conducted. I knew it had gotten ridiculous when I saw an advertisement (and a website) for an upcoming "national summit" on CER sponsored by a for-profit medical conference company, "featuring a comparative effectiveness boot camp." (Let's see now, calculating quality-adjusted life years while wearing olive-drab fatigues?) I am not making this up.

The term "comparative effectiveness research" seems to be a relatively recent coinage, but the concept has been around forever. It is usually called technology assessment. The idea is to figure out which drug, device, treatment, or diagnostic test works best for a given condition in a given population. You do that by comparing active interventions with each other, not with placebos, to produce conclusions that are useful in real-world settings.

We have well-documented geographical variation in care in the US, in terms of rates of elective surgery, costs of procedures, practice patterns in caring for patients with specific diseases—you name it. Because there are few or no corresponding variations in health outcomes, everyone thinks there must be waste in there somewhere. If we could only find it and eliminate it, we should be able to decrease costs and improve quality of care. That is where CER comes in.

The theory is that doctors and patients don't know whether talk therapy or drug treatment is better for attention deficit/hyperactivity disorder, or the best way to treat low back pain, or whether stents, surgery, or drugs are best for coronary artery disease. If only we had head-to-head trials or clever analyses of large clinical databases to compare them, we could figure this out, and the variation (and costs) would rapidly decrease. It is seen by some as no less than a panacea.

So, thought leaders have been promoting CER for the past several years, without much success. Then the huge stimulus package that Congress was considering early this year presented a golden opportunity. Finding $1.1 billion for CER was easy when the budget for the total bill was $787 billion.

Interestingly, however, there was a lot of opposition to the inclusion of funds for CER in the stimulus bill. Just before its final passage, lobbyists for drug and medical device manufacturers worked overtime to remove the funding. They ultimately failed and now deny that they were against CER. They say that they were only concerned that such research would stifle innovation and lead to government rationing of care, with the least expensive drugs and treatments being favored.

So they formed an instant grassroots organization, the Partnership to Improve Patient Care, to monitor how the CER funds are administered. Although the organization's website lists as members dozens of medical societies and disease advocacy groups, the steering committee (and presumably the funding) is dominated by the powerful "big three": the trade associations for the medical device, biotechnology, and drug manufacturers. At every CER forum I have attended they have all been there, testifying to the importance of individualized care and the need to exclude cost considerations from comparative effectiveness analyses.

It is not just the drug and device manufacturers who are against CER. Conservative commentators have accused it of denying freedom of choice to patients and coming between patients and their doctors. They see CER as the first step toward government controlled and rationed care, threatening personalized medicine.

It is no surprise that CER has become controversial. You only have to look at the history of technology assessment around the world to learn that when drugs and devices are compared, some win and some lose. The stakes are high, and no one likes to lose.

It seems to me that CER is neither the panacea that some proclaim nor the devil's work that others decry. The variation in care across the US is not just a knowledge problem. It is driven in part by lack of knowledge, but also by local traditions, fear of lawsuits, physicians' desire for personal gain, and the way our health care system is organized. Research alone will not fix all of these.

It would be a shame, though, if the constant lobbying by conservatives and the industry dilutes the focus and narrows the scope of the CER that the Department of Health and Human Services sponsors. While it won't fix everything, $1.1 billion could fund useful research and methodological advances if it is applied thoughtfully.

A committee on CER appointed by the Institute of Medicine is due to report at the end of this month. It is likely that it will come up with recommendations for specific studies and infrastructure, recommendations that should be heeded. I hope that the committee also points out that costs, when used to assess value, are an integral part of comparing the effectiveness of medical interventions. Also, they should say that none of this will make any difference unless the results of the research are actually incorporated into how we deliver care. We will not have gotten much for our billion dollars if the research is done but not applied.

BMJ, August 1, 2009

Who will pay and who will say no?

Not everyone can get what they want from the US health care reforms

We are now in a difficult period in the attempt to reform the health care "system" in the United States. Initial optimism has waned, President Obama's popularity has plummeted, and the doomsayers are hanging the burial crepe. Shades of 1994, the year of Hillary Clinton's failed attempt at health care reform.

Earlier this year there was unprecedented cooperation not only between Democrats and (some) Republicans but also within the ruling Democratic party. This has now splintered. Most of the powerful special interest groups—doctors, hospitals, big pharma, and the insurance and health plan industry—were on board as well, falling over themselves to make public concessions so as to maintain a place at the negotiating table. Sadly, those days of bonhomie are gone.

The problem is that no one is willing to give up much. Further, no one is willing to admit that someone will have to say no to the sometimes extravagant ways of the past. The hard part is still ahead, and two related issues loom especially large: paying for the new coverage, and saying no to inappropriate care.

Given that the US already spends a larger percentage of its gross domestic product on health care than any other major country and that we have large disparities in costs with few differences in outcomes, it is tempting to assume that there must be waste in there somewhere. Simply find the waste, cut it out, and bingo—enough funding emerges to cover the previously uninsured. It is not that easy, though. We got where we are because no one wanted to be told what to do: not patients, not doctors, and not health systems. So it is no small matter to rein in the spending that has gotten out of control.

One widely chanted mantra for saving money to pay for reform is to invest in putative panaceas such as preventive medicine and health information technology. The sad truth is that appropriate preventive care, though a wise investment in health, rarely actually saves money. Also, instituting electronic medical records will be enormously expensive in the short run, given our many different systems and massive need for electronic infrastructure in individual practices. There is not much money to be saved there, either. Which is why the independent Congressional Budget Office refuses to rate either prevention or health IT as offsetting the costs of new coverage.

Only tax money—such as the proposed tax increase on people with higher incomes or new taxes on health insurance benefits—will pay for the costs of covering the uninsured. Of course, both of these are risky politically.

The second issue is control. Part of the reason that US health care costs so much is that first, we don't always know the best way to treat problems and, second, when we do we don't always do it. Comparative effectiveness research is supposed to give us this kind of information, but those with special interests have worked hard to ensure that the results of such research won't have the force of law or regulation behind them. Doing this research and not enforcing the findings is silly and wasteful. Someone, some entity, has to have the power to say no.

What it all comes down to is incentives. Given our predominantly fee-for-service system, there is no getting around the fact that doing more, whether you are a doctor or a hospital, leads to more charges and thus more income. Until that basic equation is altered—by creating new systems of care and giving those systems overall responsibility for expenses for a population—we will never slow the growth of spending.

So what will we do? Some argue for smaller, piecemeal reforms that will fix a few of the obvious problems we have: tort reform to reduce malpractice lawsuits and the resulting practice of expensive "defensive medicine"; health insurance portability to ensure that people can take their coverage with them when they change jobs; better coverage of preventive care; and changes in tax policies to allow cheaper individual and group policies.

None of these, however, will change the basic incentive of do more, get more.

The dangers of the current course are that we may not get any reform at all, which would not only miss a real opportunity but ultimately bankrupt us. Or we could go part way and not get real reform that fundamentally changes the incentives and reorders the system. Or, finally, we could get "real" health care reform, which might not work, costing an enormous amount of money and not yielding corresponding increases in coverage, outcomes, and satisfaction.

Republicans are seeing blood in the water and are now working hard to kill any reform. They have no real comprehensive alternative to offer, but the public is impatient and receptive to clever negative advertising comparing health care reform to irrelevant government fiascos such as the response to Hurricane Katrina.

It is pretty close to panic time. Will we have health care reform, will we have nothing, or will we go part way? It seems to me that unless we have enough reform to cover almost everyone, create an institution that will say no when the evidence is against treatments, and change the incentives so that they are aligned for appropriate rather than just more care, we will have accomplished nothing.

BMJ, September 12, 2009

The gatekeeper and the wizard, redux
An Olde World fairy tale,* exported to America

Once upon a time, in a country far away, lived a great wizard with wondrous healing powers. He lived in a splendid castle on a hill overlooking the city. The wizard was clever. He knew how to use magic crystals to see inside people to find out what was wrong with them, and he had magic spells and potions to treat their illnesses. When sick people came to see the wizard, he often cured them or made them feel better and live longer. For his work he was paid handsomely.

Down the hill, in a nice big house, though not as grand as the wizard's, lived a gatekeeper. An important part of her job was to decide who got to see the wizard. She was also clever, and she had magic potions as well. After all, she and the wizard had gone to the same school, though they had learned different sorts of magic after leaving it. All the people who felt poorly came to see her. For the most part the gatekeeper could tell who needed to see the wizard and who didn't. She treated most of them herself and sent a few up the hill to see the wizard. She was paid well for her work, though not nearly as well as the wizard.

In olden days there were many more gatekeepers than wizards. This made sense, because most people who felt poorly were in fact not terribly ill and were treated extremely well by gatekeepers with their potions. And the few who were very ill got to see the wizard, who used his special crystals and spells on them to good effect.

But then two things happened. First, the costs of the school for wizards and gatekeepers were greatly increased. This led many students to finish school with enormous debts. More and more decided to become wizards rather than gatekeepers because the pay was better. But that meant that now there were too few gatekeepers and too many wizards.

---

* With apologies and homage to Nigel Mathers. This is an updated and Americanized version of a series of fairy tales he published in the *BMJ* about 20 years ago (see bibliography).

The second thing that happened was that the rules were changed. Anyone who felt poorly—or even those who didn't—could go directly up the hill to see the wizard. They no longer had to stop and see the gatekeeper first. These two changes led to big trouble.

Even though wizards were excellent at treating very sick people, it turned out that gatekeepers were much better at telling who was sick and who was not. And gatekeepers charged much less for their magic. Almost everyone who saw a wizard ended up being viewed through magic crystals and treated with his spells and potions. And the wizard's powerful crystals and spells not only cost a lot, but they didn't really help people who weren't very ill. Sometimes their side effects even made people worse. Also, there were now so few gatekeepers that many people couldn't find one. Costs were out of control, lots of people couldn't afford care when they were sick, and the countryside was in an uproar.

Then a new prince came to power, young but wise.

The young prince heard the concerns of the people and gave everyone hope. He promised that everyone who felt poorly could get help. He promised to improve the care that they received, and he also promised to reduce costs. These were difficult promises to keep.

One big problem was that the prince could not change the rules by himself. To make changes he had to convince the House of Gnomes that his ideas were the best. Everyone agreed that there was a problem, but they disagreed on how to fix it. It was hard work getting a consensus, especially because the gnomes had just agreed to smelt vast piles of gold for the kingdom's coffers.

The prince and his courtiers spent most of their time and energy figuring out how to pay for more people to get care. Almost no one talked about who was delivering the care: gatekeepers or wizards. Part of their plan was to control the use of the expensive crystals and spells, and that meant sending everyone to gatekeepers first. But how were people supposed to see gatekeepers first when there weren't enough of them around and when fewer and fewer students were becoming gatekeepers? No one talked about that.

The storyteller wishes he could tell you that this fable had a happy ending, but this complicated story is not finished. We do not know yet whether everyone ends up living happily ever after or not.

BMJ, October 24, 2009

All or nothing at all?

If US health reform doesn't change coverage, costs, and quality, will it matter?

As I write this, two health reform bills are moving through the US Senate and three are in the House of Representatives. Senate leadership is meeting to combine their two bills into something that will have a chance of getting through the more conservative of the two bodies. This is looking more and more likely to succeed. The House has a similar blending task for their more liberal bills, which probably shouldn't prove too difficult.

Then the bills go to the floors of the respective chambers for passage. Finally, if they make it that far, comes the conference of all conferences: an attempt to craft a bill both houses can agree on.

Most observers feel that we are pretty close to a historic change. The question is, what would a final law look like? What reforms will remain and what will get compromised away? Will the new regulations make a difference? As Frank Sinatra famously sang, should it be all or nothing at all—or is half a love enough? Here are some thoughts on the major issues.

The problems to be addressed are well documented. We spend over $2.4 trillion annually on health care. We have more than 46 million uninsured Americans. Our population health outcomes lag the developed (and some of the developing) world. That's bad.

All of the bills would require most Americans to have health insurance or pay a penalty. People with low income, and some with middle income, would get subsidies to help them afford insurance, though the subsidies are less in the Senate Finance Committee bill than they are in either the other Senate bill or the House bills. Insurance companies would be required to cover all applicants; they could no longer deny insurance because of pre-existing conditions. That's good.

Different coverage estimates accompany the different bills. The Senate Finance Committee bill, which costs the least, leaves the most people uninsured, about 17 million after 10 years. This seems unacceptable, both for moral reasons and because ultimately it would probably lead to higher costs, as people without insurance defer care and end up with more complicated and costly problems.

All the bills require a minimum level of benefits without annual or lifetime caps, including inpatient and outpatient services and preventive care. This is good. They do, however, vary in their requirements for out-of-pocket copayments for services. Again, the Senate Finance bill costs patients the most.

One of the major battles is whether or not there will be a so-called public option—a government-sponsored (presumably low-cost) plan to compete with the private plans to keep their charges—and profits—low. One of the Senate bills and all the House bills have such a public option. The Republicans and some Democrats, backed by the very strong insurance lobby, are against it, calling it unfair competition that will ultimately drive the private sector out of business, leaving a single plan: the one sponsored by the government.

It is not clear how this issue will be resolved, as liberals insist a public option will improve care and help keep costs down and conservatives see it as the road to—gasp—socialized medicine. Possible compromises include a trigger mechanism, which would provide a safety net public plan only in states without affordable private coverage, or allowing the states to sponsor public plans if they think it necessary.

How to raise the money to pay for the new system is another contentious issue. The president and Congress are committed to a "budget neutral" law, meaning that revenues have to be found to offset its cost over the first 10 years of its existence. The new system then would have to start decreasing the deficit in subsequent years. To raise the money, the House bills tax wealthy Americans and the Senate Finance bill taxes health care industries and expensive private health insurance plans. Conservatives howl that the Senate bill would really increase the financial burden on the middle class as the taxes are passed through as increased premiums. Not good.

None of this, of course, addresses the quality of health care and changing the incentives that currently pay doctors and hospitals more only when they deliver more care, rather than when they deliver better care. This is the third part of an interconnected triad with cost and access. Costs can never be controlled if there is no check on constantly delivering more care, especially if there are more people with insurance to pay for that care. The Senate

Finance bill begins to address this issue by creating a new Medicare center to test ways to improve quality and reduce costs. That is a start. None of the bills fundamentally change the current incentive structure.

In summary, my answer to the Frank Sinatra question is that, since the current system is both morally repugnant and financially unsustainable, "all or nothing at all" is a fool's choice for reform. Whatever emerges from the Congress is likely to be better than what we have now. If it is not perfect, we'll have time to improve it. Cover (many) more people, constrain costs, and begin to figure out ways to incentivize better quality. Might not make a catchy tune, but half a love is better than none.

BMJ, January 30, 2010

US health care reform is in the waste can

Can one state's senatorial election really scuttle the whole thing?

The first piece of conventional wisdom about the race for the late Edward Kennedy's US Senate seat was that there was no chance that the Republican candidate, Scott Brown, could defeat the Massachusetts attorney general, the Democrat Martha Coakley. Massachusetts is a heavily Democratic state, it was Kennedy's seat for almost 50 years, and it was crucial for the Democrats to maintain their 60–40 advantage in the US Senate.

As everyone now knows, this conventional wisdom was wrong. In the fading days of the campaign Coakley's large lead evaporated and Brown won handily, with 53 percent of the vote.

The second bit of conventional wisdom about this race, explaining the amazing upset, was that it was a vote against President Obama's policies, especially health care reform. A perfect storm, pundits said: a weak Democratic candidate, a poorly run campaign, and voters impatient for economic recovery, all in a state that already had passed its own universal health coverage law and thus "didn't need" a new federal law.

As everyone may not know, however, the answer to whether this conventional wisdom is correct is—we don't know. And we never will. Because the outcome of the race was a foregone conclusion for so long, none of the news organizations paid for the exit polling that would have told us what motivated a large number of independents to vote Republican. Was it health reform? Economic woes? Disaffection with the overwhelmingly Democratic governance in Massachusetts? An insider running in an outsider environment? Whatever caused it, the result of this one state race has had cataclysmic implications nationally.

If you have lost track of the health care reform saga over the holidays, here is where it stood on the eve of the Massachusetts election: both houses of Congress had passed different bills, either of which would have revolutionized the US health care system. To get a bill passed in the Senate, huge and unsavory compromises had been made that benefited unions, specific states, anti-abortion advocates, and others. Daily meetings were taking place to come up with a compromise version of the two bills that would be acceptable to both houses of Congress and to the White House.

This was entirely a Democratic effort. Early attempts to involve at least a token number of Republicans failed, and both bills passed with no Republican votes. To get a final bill through the 100-member Senate the Democrats needed all 60 of their votes, because of arcane rules involving the so-called filibuster. As anyone who remembers Jimmy Stewart in *Mr. Smith Goes to Washington* knows, one senator can trump the majority by holding the floor and speaking forever. This has evolved from actually holding the floor to threatening to filibuster, and 60 votes are required to defeat it. Because any negotiated compromise on the health care bill would have to be ratified in both houses, the Massachusetts vote has had incredible repercussions.

So what happens now?

Initially some people suggested that the Democrats try to vote quickly on a compromise before the Senate seated its newest member. But even Democratic senators realized that such a move would be subverting the will of the people. Others proposed that the House of Representatives, dominated by Democrats and without a filibuster rule, should just adopt the Senate version and send it to the president for signature. Soon after the election, though, the Democratic speaker of the House, Nancy Pelosi, announced that she didn't have the votes to pass the more conservative Senate bill. A third procedural trick would use something called "reconciliation" rules to pass the bill. This strategy, which would require only a simple majority for passage, was abandoned because it only applies to matters affecting financial appropriations, and parts of the bills don't involve money.

President Obama immediately suggested that a bipartisan effort could start anew to focus on aspects of reform that all parties agreed on, such as insurance reform, cost reduction, and helping out small businesses. Cynics dubbed this proposal "health care lite," and even the president conceded that it was unlikely to happen. Republicans, sensing victory, are not interested in coming to the negotiating table. Realistically, to get insurance reforms (no exclusions on the basis of pre-existing conditions, no lifetime maximums, and so on) you have to have universal coverage. That means subsidies for those people who cannot afford care, which breaks the budget. Suddenly it isn't health care lite any more.

So does this mean that the results of a single state's senatorial election will actually derail what looked until last week to be a reasonably good chance of a major change in the US health care system? Is there any way to salvage important reform from this mess?

I think it looks very unlikely indeed. Certainly the president can make some administrative reforms in the programs he controls, such as Medicare and Medicaid, to move them aggressively toward rewarding quality rather than quantity of care. He can encourage and help other states to follow Massachusetts' lead in covering more of their citizens. He can use his bully pulpit to try to gain support for a streamlined bill that doesn't have all the special interest provisions that made the current Senate bill so odious.

But I don't think anyone is optimistic that significant health care reform will emerge this year or any time soon. We had our opportunity and we squandered it.

BMJ, April 24, 2010

Prevention and the new US health reform act

Important but overlooked benefits were snuck into the bill

Contrary to many predictions (including mine; see the previous essay), President Obama and the Democrats found the will and a tricky strategy to pass sweeping health care reform legislation. Now that the bill has been signed into law, everyone is discussing what will happen and when. Critics of all persuasions are no less active than they were before passage.

Critics from the right say that the program will do nothing to staunch the hemorrhaging of spending on health care and thus will only worsen our dire economic situation. Critics from the left say that the new law is like treating cancer with morphine: it will bring temporary relief but won't alter the root cause of the problem, which they say is the private insurance system.

To some extent, both sets of critics are right. But at this point it seems to me that the only question remaining is the same one facing Congress last month when they voted: was this bill, imperfect as it was, better than doing nothing? There were only two choices at the end of the day: pass the bill, warts and all, or do nothing, probably for decades.

I come down on the side of passage for two big reasons. The first is what the projections showed things would look like in 10 years if the current system remained unchanged: an estimated 60 million uninsured people, health care spending of almost $5 trillion a year, family insurance premiums increasing to $30,000 annually, and a Medicare trust fund that runs out of money. Pretty grim.

Second, there are real, indisputable benefits to the new law. Some were much discussed and are known to all: a dramatic increase of coverage among the uninsured, portability of plans across jobs and states, and the prohibition of denial of coverage for pre-existing conditions. Some of the features of the law, however, are not well known. They were quietly inserted when everyone's attention was diverted by "hot button" issues such as abortion, the need for a "public" plan, and individual pork-barrel provisions for the states of wavering senators.

Many of these unsung provisions are in the area of health promotion and disease prevention. Careful reading of the bill reveals a surprising and almost shockingly broad set of prevention-related changes and enhancements that span personal health care, public health, and community infrastructure.

From September 23, six months after the bill was signed, all new US health insurance policies must cover every evidence-based clinical preventive service—screening tests, immunizations, and counseling interventions—at no cost to beneficiaries. This eliminates deductibles and copayments, which have been shown to be disincentives to the delivery of preventive care. Services covered will include all preventive care recommended by the US Preventive Services Task Force. Many health plans already made these services available without charge, but this provision standardizes future coverage for everyone who is insured.

There is a loophole to this provision. Only "new" policies are covered. Are policies "new" when they are renewed each year? Probably not. It will be up to the regulators to define new, and this could lead to delays in implementation of the coverage. Medicare patients won't face delays, however. Almost every American age 65 or older and younger people who are disabled will get this benefit without the loophole, starting January 1, 2011.

Another new Medicare benefit is the expansion of the single "welcome to Medicare" wellness visit to an annual preventive check-up. All Medicare patients will be entitled to a no-cost annual visit that includes a health risk assessment, creation of a personalized prevention plan, and appropriate screening tests and immunizations, effective from January 1.

Medicaid beneficiaries, whose number will be dramatically increased by the new law, will also see an increase in preventive care coverage. In addition, pregnant women with Medicaid will be entitled to coverage for smoking cessation programs from October 1. The states, which administer Medicaid, will also receive grants to provide incentives to Medicaid beneficiaries to enlist in comprehensive and proved wellness programs. Funds to evaluate these programs are provided.

Employers, who provide most health insurance in the US, are also included in the prevention benefits of the new law, especially relating to employee wellness programs. Many large companies already offer these, and from 2011 small businesses can apply to a $200 million fund for grants to subsidize their wellness programs. The law also increases, from 20 percent to 30 percent, the allowable premium discount that employers may offer to employees who participate in wellness programs. A 10-state demonstration is authorized to evaluate employer wellness programs from 2014.

Finally, a $5 billion federal prevention and public health fund is created to pay for community infrastructure, such as bike paths, playgrounds, sidewalks, and hiking trails, to increase physical activity and build healthier communities. Also, chain restaurants will be required to provide full nutritional information on their menus to allow their customers to see just how many calories that Big Mac contains (540, if you're wondering).

All in all, in addition to providing for health care coverage for more Americans, the health reform act should also result in improvements in health promotion and disease prevention. Even if costs are not cut, we will likely be purchasing improved health with the dollars we spend.

BMJ, April 30, 2011

PCORI: odd name, important job, potential trouble

Research institute mandated by health reform begins work in the spotlight

In the last few years, there has been much debate in the US about comparative effectiveness research (CER), defined by the Institute of Medicine as "the generation and synthesis of evidence that compares the benefits and harms of alternative methods to prevent, diagnose, treat, and monitor a clinical condition or to improve the delivery of care." According to the IOM, the idea is "to assist consumers, clinicians, purchasers, and policy makers to make informed decisions that will improve health care at both the individual and population levels."

CER first vaulted into the news here when Congress dedicated $1.1 billion to it as part of the fiscal stimulus package passed in 2009, at the height of the recession.* The Department of Health and Human Services, through NIH and the Agency for Healthcare Research and Quality, quickly disbursed those funds to sponsor research and research infrastructure development to improve medical decisions and clinical outcomes by comparing various drugs, treatments, and other interventions.

Some critics, often pharmaceutical or medical device manufacturers, warned that CER would disadvantage certain new and expensive treatments that head-to-head trials found were only marginally more effective than cheaper, currently available treatments. Other critics, mainly conservatives in the US, were worried that a slavish adherence to CER findings would lead to rationing, inhibiting "individual choice" and dooming individuals to receive only treatments that government bureaucrats chose for them.

Despite these concerns, the government role in CER did not end with the stimulus package. Thus was born the Patient-Centered Outcomes Research Institute. Affectionately known as PCORI, it was initially a little-noticed provision of the Affordable Care Act, the health reform legislation. It established PCORI as an independent research institute to sponsor CER.

---

* See page 102.

PCORI is funded generously, mainly from a tap on health insurance premiums. By 2013, it will have a budget of about half a billion dollars a year to spend on research and research dissemination.

This sounds great, right? A well-funded independent institute to do CER to improve care and reduce costs. But like most things in government, and certainly much in the Affordable Care Act, it is not quite that straightforward.

First, a search of the enabling legislation fails to find CER mentioned in it at all. Instead, it has been replaced by something called "comparative *clinical* effectiveness research." This is meant to restrict PCORI-sponsored research to noneconomic assessments. In fact, PCORI-funded work is specifically proscribed from using quality-adjusted life years or other such measures common in cost-effectiveness analyses. Further, the HHS secretary cannot use the results of PCORI-funded research to determine or deny coverage or reimbursement for health care services.

Second, there is PCORI's odd name. What is "patient-centered outcomes research," anyway? Why not just call it the CER institute? This, it turns out, is a legacy of concerns that CER will only find "on average" what works best for most people in large trials, thereby discriminating against individuals, especially individuals with disabilities or guarded prognoses. Hence, patient-centered.

Organizations such as the Partnership to Improve Patient Care, an Astroturf (fake) grass-roots group whose steering committee includes the major lobbyists for drug and device manufacturers, show up at every board meeting to make sure PCORI is "communicating results rather than setting centralized coverage decisions, addressing the full range of information gaps that matter to patients, addressing differences in individual patient needs, and supporting continued medical advances." Translation? Supporting expensive new drugs that extend life for a few months at huge cost.

Third, creating a new research organization the size of a small NIH institute out of nothing is not a trivial matter. Ask the people at the UK's controversial National Institute for Health and Clinical Excellence (NICE). The Affordable Care Act only mandated the appointment of a governing board for PCORI, and they have had the immense job of creating a full-fledged research institute overnight in open view of a critical public. Not an easy task.

So far, the PCORI board has worked diligently to craft bylaws, hire a staff, and begin work. They first have to figure out what patient-centered outcomes research is. Then they have to decide what research to fund and how to go about it. While the board has not actually spent a dime yet on research, this hasn't stopped the *Wall Street Journal* and other conservative voices from sniping at them as part of their campaign against CER: "comparative effectiveness isn't about informing choices. It's really about taking away options." Despite the posting of PCORI board member biographies on the web and the webcasting of their public meetings, the *Journal* demands to know "who these people are and what they favor."

Partially crippled by its wacky name and its inability to sponsor cost-effectiveness research, PCORI is treading a treacherous road toward a noble goal. I hope they are not distracted by the special interest clamor and conservative clap-trap. CER is not a panacea, but it has real potential to improve care and decrease costs. If head-to-head trials help us compare treatments and treatment systems for common problems, we can improve quality and safety. If just a few of the expensive boondoggles we fervently believe in are exposed and expunged, CER can rationalize (not ration) care and pay for itself. It would be nice if everyone would just leave them alone and let them get on with it.

5

Personal Stories and Ethical Issues

"I am always at a loss to know how much to believe of my own stories."

—Washington Irving, 1783–1859

The essays in this final section are based on my own personal experiences, which either led to the commentary or seemed to illuminate a specific issue well. The lone exception to this is the first piece, on the physician's role in capital punishment. I thought it was an interesting and complex ethical issue, with good arguments on both sides of whether doctors and other health professionals should assist the state in killing people. I have had no personal experience with capital punishment.

Otherwise, though, my medical background has provided direct experience related to all of the commentaries in this section. Flying on a plane is something we all do, and it is a uniquely isolated environment if one becomes ill. I have been called on to help sick passengers, and I spent some time looking into the statistics about illnesses on planes.

When a Maryland mother started marketing a placebo pill for children, it reminded me of when I prescribed placebos as a medical intern. I thought it was somewhat justifiable then, but I can see no reason for parents to give their children little red sugar pills. I could not resist attacking this as a very bad idea.

One commentary, on the ethics of doctors receiving gifts from drug companies, brought back memories of gifts I had received (or rejected) as a medical student and resident. Another, on concerns about honesty in claiming authorship of medical journal articles, reminded me of discussions and negotiations I have had about whose name should go on a journal article and in what order. I was shocked, though, to learn, as a by-product of the Vioxx controversy investigation, the extent to which drug companies literally bought and sold authorship of articles in prestigious medical journals.

Two commentaries in this section are centered on my mother. The first recounts my efforts to sign her up for Medicare's complicated new prescription drug benefit. It was a humbling experience. The second, which is the last essay in this book, was written a week after my mother died. It summarizes the many things I learned from her in her final years about health and health care.

BMJ, March 3, 2007

Killing me softly

Can the prevention of suffering justify the involvement of doctors in capital punishment?

Ninety-four percent of the world's executions occur in four countries. China executes the most people, at least 1,000 and maybe as many as 8,000 a year. Iran and Saudi Arabia are next, with around 100. The United States is fourth. In 2006 we killed 53 convicted murderers, down from 60 in 2005. In the 30 years since 1977, when the US Supreme Court moratorium on capital punishment ended, about 1,000 Americans have been executed, a third of them in Texas, the rest in 33 other states.

Putting someone to death is not easy or pretty. As Elizabeth Weil pointed out in a recent *New York Times Magazine* article on the subject, each time a new method of capital punishment has been introduced it has been because the then current method was found to be barbaric and uncivilized. Death by hanging can lead to a dangling, kicking, prolonged struggle, or a gruesome rope beheading. Firing squads are hard to control and sometimes inaccurate, leaving the victims alive. Gas chambers take a long time, and death by suffocation is not attractive. Electrocution commonly results in grotesquely charred flesh and occasionally in flaming heads and other body parts. Sometimes it doesn't work.

Which is why we now do virtually all of our executions in the US by lethal injection. Nice and clean, sterile setting, looks like a hospital. People dressed in white, alcohol swabs, cardiac monitors, intravenous lines. When all goes right, three quick intravenous injections—sodium thiopental to put the condemned to sleep, a paralyzing agent so as not to offend the witnesses with any gasps or jerky movements, and potassium chloride to stop the heart—and in a few minutes, a "humane" and certifiable death.

But things don't always go right. Several recent widely publicized fiascos have made that clear. In Florida, poorly trained technicians placed two IVs in the arms of a condemned man named Angel Diaz. Neither one was in a vein. The potassium infused subcutaneously, causing chemical burns. His painful death took more than 30 minutes, during most of which he was awake and speaking. This led Governor Jeb Bush to declare a moratorium on executions in Florida until they can figure out a better way to execute the 372 (!) others on death row there.

And that, unfortunately, is where the medical profession comes in. If lethal injection is going to be done correctly, you need someone with medical expertise to do it, or at least to train the people who do it and to supervise them. The US constitution specifies that no "cruel or unusual punishment" is allowed. Leaving aside for a minute the argument that capital punishment itself is cruel, certainly making people suffer needlessly is.

Surgeon Atul Gawande interviewed four doctors and a nurse who had participated in executions for a compelling article in the *New England Journal of Medicine* last year. Some of them stated that if capital punishment is legal, then executions should be done competently, and that means with medical supervision. One of the doctors compared executions to other end of life situations. When a patient is dying it is up to a physician to make sure the death is as pain-free and comfortable as possible, whether death is caused by nature or the state. Some of the participating doctors were state employees, whose job it was to care for prisoners. The men and women on death row were their patients.

Others argue that there can be no doctor-patient relationship between the doctor who facilitates an execution and the person to be executed, because the doctor is not putting the "patient's" welfare first. Since at least 1980, the policy of the American Medical Association has been that physicians may not participate in executions because they are members of "a profession dedicated to preserving life when there is hope of doing so." Does that take precedence over preventing the suffering that will occur if doctors are *not* involved in lethal injections?

Other countries don't seem to have the same problem figuring out how to execute their criminals. Weil wrote that China has a "suite of hyper-efficient lethal-injection vans that drive around the provinces carrying trained teams that execute the condemned." No muss, no fuss.

And that is the real problem: we don't want a mess. We want these evil people to disappear, to be dead, but most of us don't want to feel bad about how they died. In the more remote past, hangings were public; the citizenry attended and saw everything. Now we do it in secret, we can't bear to watch, and we want it to be painless.

Lots of reasons are advanced against capital punishment: it is immoral, it reduces the state to the level of the killer, and it is irreversible if we find we have made a mistake. But if there is even one killer, one crime that is so heinous to "deserve" a capital sentence, we have to accept that killing people is not pleasant. Sometimes it is going to go wrong and we will feel bad. If we cannot accept that then we should not be killing people on behalf of the state—with or without the help of doctors.

NPR, November 15, 2007

Medicare Part D signup blues

Way more complicated than it needs to be

I don't have Medicare (yet) but my mother does, so I offered to sign her up online. Shouldn't be too hard, I thought. I'm a reasonably smart guy. I'm good with computers. And I'm a doctor, so I know the lingo.

I knew what to do: gather up her Medicare card and list of medicines, go to Medicare's website, enter all the requested data, and pick the plan that would give her the best deal on prescriptions. Guess what: it is not that simple.

I typed in her zip code and found that no fewer than 52 plans were available. They all had different premium prices, deductible levels, and coverage policies. These are displayed for you in endless tables on your screen. These tables don't tell the whole story, however. Your best deal also depends on the number and type of drugs you're taking, whether they are available generically, and how each plan ranks your drugs in a four-tiered pricing scheme.

All of this is, of course, is superimposed on the ebb and flow of drug benefits through the year that Congress mandated. You remember hearing about this. First, there's a deductible period, when you pay everything. Then, the plan pays a lot for a few months. Then you fall into the so-called "doughnut hole" and you pay everything. Finally, if your drugs cost more than $4000, the plan starts paying again. Simple, huh?

If you think this is a scheme that cries out for a spreadsheet, you're right. Because what you really want to know after you jump through all these hoops is, what will each plan cost me for a year's worth of my drugs? To give them credit, the folks at Medicare have provided an online calculator that will more or less tell you just that. Only after you answer a bunch of questions and after you enter all the drugs and dosages, of course. Assuming it is working, which it wasn't the first time I tried.

Even a list of drug plans ranked by their total cost doesn't tell you which one to choose. Should you take a program that pays for drugs in the doughnut hole in case your doctor adds some expensive medicines during the year? What is the relative importance of having a lower deductible versus lower monthly premiums? And so forth.

All of which is to ask: what in the world was Congress thinking when they created this mess? If a computer-savvy doctor is having so much trouble picking the best program for his mother, how are the vast majority of Medicare patients ever going to pick their plans wisely?

Who could possibly benefit from this arcane set of rules and regulations? Hint: it's the same people who lobbied for this crazy system 2 years ago. The same ones who raised premium costs an average of 27 percent for 2008. You guessed it: it's the insurance companies and the drug companies.

BMJ, May 3, 2008

Who wrote that article?

The latest revelations about ghost authorship of journal articles are truly frightening

Authorship issues are a common obsession of medical journal editors. They fuss about them a great deal, fretting about who contributed what to a paper, who was responsible for the work and its conclusions, and what should qualify a contributor to assume the august title of "author." The quantity and, to a lesser extent, the quality of authored publications have a lot to do with who gets promoted in academia, who gets tenured, and who gets jobs at prestigious universities. So naturally there is a great desire among academics to get their names on as many papers as possible, preferably at the head of the (often lengthy) list of authors.

I don't think anyone in the outside world cares much about all of this. It's easy to make fun of the competition, quibbling, and controversy surrounding authorship by reminding everyone of the old saw that the reason the politics are so intense in academic medicine is that the stakes are so low. After all, who is really harmed if a few old men's names are gratuitously added to a list of authors or if a research assistant's contributions go uncredited?

The stakes are raised substantially, though, when the drug industry becomes involved. In support of their products, drug companies sponsor carefully orchestrated campaigns to pass off sympathetic, if not biased, research and review articles as the work of academic scientists rather than of their own or contracted employees. Ghost authorship takes on a new meaning when health communication companies write papers on contract, recruit prestigious authors for them, and then disappear from view. Former *BMJ* editor Richard Smith, in his 2006 book *The Trouble with Medical Journals*, recounts a story of an employee of one such firm bragging that she was a leading author of articles in prestigious medical journals despite never having her name appear on the papers.

I knew that ghostwriting had been documented at rates of between 6 percent and 15 percent of various types of medical journal articles and that "gift authorship" is even more common. But I never really appreciated either the depth of the problem or its pervasiveness until two weeks ago. The litigation surrounding the drug company Merck and its pain reliever Vioxx (rotecoxib) led to the public release of millions of company documents. In a shocking case study of about 250 of these documents published in *JAMA* on April 16, Joseph Ross and colleagues matched up drafts of company-authored research articles and contract-authored review articles with the subsequently published papers. Comparing the lists of authors on the draft and final versions of these almost 100 papers is chilling.

Although we've known about these practices for years, it is creepy to actually see the title pages of succeeding drafts of articles, first with only drug company authors and then with one to three recruited academic authors' names magically appearing at the top. In the series looked at in the *JAMA* article, the first author of 16 of 20 reviewed research articles changed from a Merck author to an external, academically affiliated investigator between the draft and the published version.

The findings for review articles are even worse. At least in the research studies, the Merck authors' names remained on the paper. Most of the review articles in the study were ghostwritten by contract communication companies and "edited" (for an honorarium) by external academics who were then given sole authorship. The *JAMA* article reprints an e-mail from a contractor in which the progress of eight review articles is communicated to Merck staff, complete with article title, intended journal, and desired (external) author. Seven of the eight review articles were subsequently published. Also reprinted is a contract showing that the going rate for one of these review articles in 2001 was just under $24,000.

It is not being overly dramatic to say that public trust in clinical research, in the medical journals that report research, and in medicine in general is at stake here. Unless we can be reasonably certain that research results and review articles are unbiased, we can't know whether doctors are giving—and the public is getting—correct advice and care. And unless we know who wrote the articles and paid for the research, we can't completely assess the work for bias.

What can be done? Scandals like this will presumably help discourage such practices. Proper disclosure of research funding and authorship helps a lot, allowing readers to know who is behind the work. External statistical input and impartial peer review help prevent and identify problems too.

Do we need to go even further? Since so much drug research is funded by the drug industry, it is unlikely that a prohibition of such funding is feasible. Maybe journals should refuse review articles from authors with any support from the industry. This was done by some journals a few years ago, but the policy was reversed.

Unfortunately, no matter how many rules and regulations are in place, this is ultimately a matter of trust. Liars and unscrupulous companies will continue to get away with these practices some of the time despite everyone's best efforts. It is a depressing thought.

NPR, May 12, 2008

Aesculapius on a plane

What happens when there is a medical emergency in the air?

If you fly a lot, you have likely been on a plane when they asked if there was a doctor on board. On a flight some years ago, I responded to such a call. After showing my credentials to a flight attendant, I was taken to see a young man who seemed drowsy and couldn't focus.

"What's wrong?" I asked. No response.

"Do you have any medical problems?" No response.

"Do you take any medicines?" No response.

Luckily, his traveling companion gave us an important clue: the passenger had diabetes. His seatmate had found a vial of insulin and a syringe in the passenger's travel bag and was urging the crew—and me—to administer it.

That would have been a big mistake, of course, maybe even a fatal one, given the relative risks of hypoglycemia and hyperglycemia. The standard treatment for an unresponsive patient with diabetes is to give them something with glucose in it first, to see if their problem is low blood sugar, hypoglycemia. If their blood sugar is low, the glucose will help. If it is already too high—hyperglycemia—a little more glucose won't hurt much. But the opposite isn't true. If a patient's blood sugar is already low, because of too much diabetes medicine or insulin, then a further shot of insulin could lead to hypoglycemic coma or even death.

So, it was with some conviction that I said something like, "Hold it. Put the insulin away and let's try some orange juice first." It worked. After a while the patient woke up and felt better. It turned out that he had taken some insulin just before the flight, anticipating a meal that hadn't come soon enough.

The American news media breathlessly reported a story recently about a woman with diabetes and heart disease who died on a flight from Haiti to New York, despite being attended to by the flight crew and several doctors who happened to be passengers on the flight. Her family alleged that the medical equipment on the plane was not in working order and that her initial complaints had been ignored by the crew. The airline stated that all equipment functioned properly and that she had been treated appropriately by the crew and doctors. The plane was not diverted while en route and her dead body was removed once they reached New York.

The event raised all manner of questions about medical care on commercial airplanes. Who is responsible for responding to medical emergencies in the air? What equipment and medications are available? Who decides whether treatment is necessary and what, if any, to administer? When is diversion of the flight appropriate?

Serious in-flight medical events are uncommon, occurring in between 1 in 10,000 and 1 in 40,000 passengers. Because there are so many people flying these days, however, such emergencies actually happen somewhere several times every day. It has been estimated that hundreds of patients die each year while flying, almost always from a pre-existing condition.

Some airline emergencies are new problems, like vasovagal reactions—fainting—upon standing after sitting for a long time, or gastrointestinal disorders. But most are exacerbations of known chronic conditions, like my patient's diabetes or, more commonly, heart or lung diseases. It is worth remembering that the cabin air pressure during a flight is equivalent to that at an altitude of 5,000 to 8,000 feet on the ground. This may be low enough to cause hypoxia and breathlessness in patients with cardiac or pulmonary disease. Often problems arise because needed medications have been checked in baggage instead of carried on the flight, especially those for angina or asthma.

For cardiac arrest, flight attendants are certified in cardiopulmonary resuscitation. Oxygen is available, and planes are now required to carry automatic external defibrillators. Flight staff are trained in their use as well. There is also a complete medical kit on board most airliners, which can be opened and used under the supervision of a medical professional, either on the plane or by radio from the ground. It contains a stethoscope, blood pressure cuff, intravenous equipment, and common oral and intravenous medications.

It is estimated that between a half and three-quarters of all flights have, by chance, a doctor, nurse, or paramedic on board. If they volunteer, they're asked to assess the problem and stabilize the affected passenger. Occasionally they advise the pilot about whether the flight needs to be diverted so that the patient can get treatment sooner. They can also consult by radio with medical staff on the ground who are on call for such events.

In the United States, Canada, and the United Kingdom, doctors are not required to volunteer to help patients in distress, but several European countries and Australia do impose a legal duty to assist. Most countries have "good Samaritan" laws protecting doctors from legal liability if they give good faith care at a level commensurate with their training.

The most important advice for all patients is to carry their medications with them in their carry-on bag. Those at increased risk for an event that might leave them unconscious—such as diabetes, epilepsy, coronary artery disease, and severe hypertension—should travel with a companion or wear a medical identification bracelet. Persons with compromised breathing should consider arranging for supplemental oxygen on board when making their reservations.

Doctors flying on commercial airplanes should not be afraid to render care when called on. The most important contributions doctors can make are, as always, a careful history and assessment. It is not their job to take control, but rather to serve as advisors to the crew and, on occasion, to medical staff on the ground.

BMJ, June 14, 2008

Placebo pills for children

A deeply bad idea

Another trend has begun in America. This time it is placebo pills for kids.

On June 1, a company called Efficacy Brands (I am not making this up) put cherry-flavored sugar tablets on sale on the web. The company was started by a mother with three young children, who has appeared on the morning television shows to publicize her inspiration. For just under $6, you can order a bottle of these pills to "treat" children when real medicine isn't appropriate and a hug and a kiss aren't enough. The pill is called Obecalp—placebo spelled backwards. How clever is that?

I first became aware of the power of placebos 30 years ago when I was a medical intern in a large US urban hospital. Our pharmacy stocked two "special" painkilling drugs, available by a doctor's prescription only. One came in a brilliant red capsule and the other was deep purple. The interns were instructed that these pills were for people who abused pain medications and were to be dispensed with care—and with a good story. It turned out that the red one was aspirin and the purple one was Tylenol (acetaminophen), although you couldn't find those exact words anywhere on the labels, which had (in small print) the obscure generic constituents of the medications. And sure enough, I had a number of patients who said to me that they simply had to have that red pill, or that purple one, insisting that it was the only thing that took their pain away.

If it is ever ethical to use a placebo—and I'm not sure that it is—this is an example of when it might be appropriate: helping someone with a chronic problem, using a medicine with proven efficacy, and one that is not too dangerous. Further, it was to be given without completely lying about what was in it. This meets many, but not all, of the criteria set out in a recent *BMJ* article offering guidance for prescribing placebos.

In a randomized controlled trial in the same issue, Ted Kaptchuk and colleagues cleverly deconstructed the components of the placebo effect. They showed that an important part of how placebos work is the patient-clinician relationship. In their study, the response rate went from 44 percent to 62 percent when the clinician added "warmth, attention, and confidence" when delivering placebo acupuncture to treat the symptoms of irritable bowel syndrome. It is a great demonstration of what psychiatrist and GP trainer Michael Balint called the effect of the "doctor as drug."

Doctors know that we have this personal drug available, and good doctors dispense it wisely and effectively. The power of reassurance, empathy, and confidence can go a long way toward helping patients with any number of complaints, and of course parents have a similar power to comfort and even heal their children.

While I can think of situations in which it might be appropriate for doctors to administer a placebo pill, I can't say the same for parents. The problems are numerous.

First, who are we treating here, children or their parents? If placebos are to work, the patients need to believe in them. Are doctors thus going to dispense these pills to the parents for their children, without telling them it is an inactive substance? Or is it left to the parents to determine that it is appropriate to trick their children into believing they are getting real medicine to help them?

Second, what will happen when the children become adolescents and find out that they were being sold a pill of goods, so to speak? Such a discovery cannot be good for their trust in their parents, which is often at a nadir at that age anyway.

Third, if parents use placebos to comfort their children, what are they teaching them? That pills are the answer for all our aches and pains? Perhaps for all our other problems too? Not advisable.

Finally, what makes us think that kids actually want medicine? If all children are like my three, who are now all teenagers, they won't take medicine when they are little, and they don't want it when they are big either.

And I don't buy the argument that giving a child a placebo pill is just like putting a Band-Aid on a scratch: we know it doesn't make any difference, but we tell the kids that it does. Sure, there are kids who end up wanting a colorful bandage for every possible ache and injury, but I have never seen an adult addicted to Band-Aids. I have seen many adults who want a pill for every ill.

All in all, a placebo pill for children seems like a deeply bad idea, however well intentioned. Kids who are in pain, or sick, but don't require real medicine need someone to give them a hug or a kiss or, if a treat is indicated, maybe a piece of candy. But they don't need a sugar pill, and they certainly don't need to be deceived into thinking that it is the pill's magic, not Mom's or Dad's, that helped them feel better.

BMJ, May 9, 2009

No gifts, please, we're doctors

New recommendations from the Institute of Medicine are broad and deep

When I began medical school in 1974, I was a fanatic about pharmaceutical industry gifts to students. The drug companies gave us all manner of tools for doctors—reflex hammers, stethoscopes, the works, nicely branded with their logos—and I was one of the few who rejected them all. In particular, I remember several beautifully illustrated books on anatomy, or maybe it was histology, that were actually required texts for one of our courses. I couldn't believe that the school would allow what I considered advertising into the curriculum.

Time passed, and I became less and less vigilant. By the time I was a resident I was enjoying pizza parties sponsored by the "detail men" (drug salesmen). As a young GP I was happy to prowl the exhibits at meetings and pick up the ever more impressive gifts to be had for listening to a pitch for their latest blockbuster: a computer mouse, an engraved pen, lots of fancy small flashlights, and plenty of samples for personal use. The detail men were now mostly women and they were always happy to fix us up with some antibiotics or antacids for the family or a case of infant formula for the new baby at home. No quid pro quo, just happy to help out.

I was reminded of all of this while reading the press coverage about the new Institute of Medicine report *Conflict of Interest in Medical Research, Education, and Practice*. Most of the newspaper and television news stories on it focused on the report's recommendation that doctors no longer accept items of material value from drug and device companies. The *New York Times* called it a "scolding report" and a "stinging indictment of many of the most common means by which drug and device makers endear themselves to doctors." It seems that the image of doctors stuffing their pockets with trinkets particularly resonated with the public and the press.

Gifts are only one of many issues that the report covers, however. Although they are a big problem—companies still spend billions on them— the most impressive thing about the report is its breadth. As the title only begins to suggest, the committee evaluated and made recommendations about conflicts of interest in biomedical research, medical education, clinical practice guideline creation, medical practice, and medical institutions. The recommended actions target everyone from medical students to deans, including drug and device companies, the National Institutes of Health, practicing doctors, medical societies, and the US Congress as well.

The report has depth as well as breadth. For instance, transparency in funding sources is an important beginning but not the end of what needs to be done. Simply disclosing conflicts is an "essential but insufficient element of policy." Rather than the current practice of medical journals simply listing competing interests and then declaring victory, the report recommends that conflicts be prohibited or eliminated at every possible level. The primary interest of the activity—whether research integrity, medical education quality, or patient welfare—is not to be unduly influenced by secondary interests such as financial gain or professional advancement. So researchers who have financial interests in drugs or devices should not be allowed to participate in human research related to their interests. Academic staff should not present lectures sponsored by the industry; nor should they serve on guideline committees dealing with drugs or devices for which they have received consulting funds. Finally, practicing doctors should not attend courses sponsored by the industry or accept funds from drug companies to serve on speakers' bureaus.

The case of free distribution of drug samples to doctors is a particularly challenging one. Some doctors insist that these samples are an important way to get needed drugs to needy patients. When I was in practice we had a whole closet full of them. What evidence there is indicates that most samples are in fact expensive brand name drugs that end up in the hands of patients who are not poor. They influence doctors' prescribing patterns and the types of refills requested by patients. That certainly squares with what happened to the drugs in our samples closet.

The government has a role as well. The report recommends that it create a national reporting system for tracking industry payments to doctors that can be cross-checked with doctors' declarations to journals, hospitals, and practices. The government could also require that all institutions establish policies on conflicts of interest and fund research in this area as well.

Reports such as this from the Institute of Medicine come out all the time, and they vary widely in their influence. Usually they make a splash on launch and then quickly sink into obscurity. Very occasionally, as with the reports on medical errors and patient safety, they are hugely influential and literally change the medical world. It may be too much to hope that the report on conflicts of interest will have that much effect. It covers an important problem comprehensively, though. It offers innovative as well as traditional recommendations. If most of them were adopted, they just might make an important difference across research, education, and health care.

BMJ, June 12, 2010

What I learned from Mom

A personal view of aging in the American health care system

My mother died on May 22 at age 86. She had Alzheimer's disease, congestive heart failure, and probably a small stroke at the end. She fell twice in her last year, causing two debilitating fractures.

In caring for her and arranging for her care I learned a lot that I should have already known.

The lessons began after my father died 8 years ago. It took a year or so, after some financial decisions had worked to her disadvantage, for my sister and me to realize that my mother was not really capable of managing her fiscal affairs. The lesson here was not her inability; rather, it was the vital and complementary contributions of life partners. She helped my father through his declining health, and he kept track of the finances.

Although I spend a lot of time railing about the crazy US health care system, I never got an up-close, personal view of what our elderly have to deal with until 3 years ago. I told my mother then that I would be happy to go online and pick a Medicare prescription drug plan for her. I got a list of her drugs and logged on to www.Medicare.gov. It was unbelievably complex. There were dozens of plans to choose from, each with different deductibles and copayment rules; each with payment schedules for her drugs; and each with different rules for the dread "doughnut hole" of no coverage. It was a nightmare. Here I was, a doctor with decent computer skills, and I was baffled. What were they thinking when they designed this?

I also learned from my mother what a sad, cruel disease Alzheimer's is. She did not even have severe Alzheimer's, but she had lost her short-term memory. This made it very difficult to be around her, as she was constantly asking the same questions over and over and over. She called us multiple times during the day and night repeating a question or concern. We were often angry at her, and (more importantly) she was always anxious.

Her Alzheimer's also meant that she was constantly disoriented in her final round of transfers to hospital, rehabilitation, assisted living, and back to hospital again. She usually had no idea where she was or why. What I learned from this was not how Alzheimer's affects individuals; rather it was how poorly institutions (especially acute care hospitals) do at informing staff about patients' disabilities. Time and again I would ask a new doctor or nurse—who had previously reviewed her chart—how my mother was doing. They would reply "she's confused today," or "she's not a very good historian."

Well, of course she's not a very good historian, she has Alzheimer's disease! My wife, who is not a doctor, asked how it was possible that "Alzheimer's disease—confused" was not stamped at the top of her medical records in big red letters. Good question.

My mother's last year demonstrated once again how dangerous falls can be to the well-being of elderly people with reduced vision, agility, and bone mineral density. Her first fall, resulting in a fractured pelvis, slowed her down for a while, though she was soon walking with a walker and participating in her usual activities. Her second fall caused a comminuted femur fracture.* It was the initiating event in the downward spiral ending in her death.

Another important lesson was how difficult it is to ensure continuity of care across multiple care settings. She would be discharged from the hospital on one dosage of diuretics for her heart failure. Somehow, when she got to her long-term care facility, despite correct transfer orders and an intrusive doctor for a son, her meds got confused and she received too little medicine, resulting in reaccumulation of fluid and readmission to the hospital. The lesson I learned was not that individuals were at fault, but that systems failed to protect her.

None of this is to say that my mother did not benefit from the hard work and kindness of many caring professionals. She did. But it is not fun and not very rewarding (in either an emotional or financial sense) to work in long-term care. It is a big challenge to recruit, train, and motivate people to do nursing assistant work. In the US we have a huge nursing shortage that is obvious to anyone who has a family member in an acute or chronic care setting.

The final lesson my mother taught me was about end of life care. It was very hard for me, as the family doctor in both senses of the term, to figure out how much care was enough. The parade of specialists assured us they

---

* A complicated break of the thigh bone into several pieces.

could fix her individual problems—tap her pleural effusion, diurese her edema,* and bypass her feeding problems with a tube. The real question, of course, was not whether they could do any or all of these things, but whether they should. Would it help her symptomatically or lead to a meaningful recovery?

In the end, she died peacefully, and we think comfortably, of no particular problem, or perhaps from all of them. I learned from my mother when the end had come, and of course so much more.

Thanks, Mom. God bless.

---

* Remove fluid that had accumulated in her lungs and legs.

Bibliography

Following are some of the sources used in writing the commentaries in this book as well as all the works referred to in the individual essays.

Great health care, guaranteed (page 3)

Abelson, R. In bid for better care, surgery with a warranty. New York Times [Internet]. 2007 May 17 [cited 2011 Jul 21]. Available from: http://www.nytimes.com/2007/05/17/business/17quality.html?_r=2

Committee on Quality of Health Care in America, Institute of Medicine. Crossing the quality chasm: a new health system for the 21st century. Washington: National Academy Press; 2001.

Committee on Quality of Health Care in America, Institute of Medicine. To err is human: building a safer health system. Washington: National Academy Press; 1999.

Retail health clinics: threat or promise? (page 6)

Bohmer R. The rise of in-store clinics—threat or opportunity? New England Journal of Medicine. 2007;356:765-8. PubMed PMID: 17314334.

Sullivan D. Retail health clinics are rolling your way. Family Practice Management. 2006 May;13(5):65-72.

CAM to the rescue (page 9)

Colquhoun D. Should NICE evaluate complementary and alternative medicine? No. BMJ. 2007 Mar 8;334:507. doi:10.1136/bmj.39122 .551250.BE.

Eisenberg DM, Davis RB, Ettner SL, Appel S, Wilkey S, Van Rompay M, et al. Trends in alternative medicine use in the United States, 1990-1997: results of a follow-up national survey. JAMA. 1998;280:1569-75. PubMed PMID: 9820257.

Franck L, Chantler C, Dixon M. Should NICE evaluate complementary and alternative medicine? Yes. BMJ. 2007 Mar 8;334:506. doi:10.1136/bmj .39122.512211.BE.

Shekelle PG, Morton SC, Suttorp MJ, Buscemi N, Friesen C. Challenges in systematic reviews of complementary and alternative medicine topics. Annals of Internal Medicine. 2005;142:1042-7.

Paying for promising but unproven technologies (page 12)

Chalkidou K, Hoy A, Littlejohns P. Making a decision to wait for more evidence: when the National Institute for Health and Clinical Excellence recommends a technology only in the context of research. Journal of the Royal Society of Medicine. 2007;100:453-460.

Pearson SD, Miller FG, Emanuel EJ. Medicare's requirement for research participation as a condition of coverage. Is it ethical? JAMA. 2006;296(8): 988-91. doi: 10.1001/jama.296.8.988.

Tunis SR, Pearson SD. Coverage options for promising technologies: Medicare's 'coverage with evidence development.' Health Affairs. 2006 Sept;25(5):1218-30. doi: 10.1377/hlthaff.25.5.1218.

Waiting for the genetic revolution (page 15)

EGAPP Working Group. Testing for cytochrome P450 polymorphisms in adults with nonpsychotic depression treated with selective serotonin reuptake inhibitors. Genetics in Medicine. 2007 Dec;9(12):819-825. doi: 10.1097/GIM.0b013e31815bf9a3.

Separating medical truths from fiction (page 18)

Vreeman RC, Carroll AE. Medical myths. BMJ. 2007 Dec 22-29;335:1288-9. doi:10.1136/bmj.39420.420370.25.

Testing errors in the doctor's office (page 20)

Hickner J, Graham DG, Elder NC, Brandt E, Emsermann CB, Dovey S, Phillips R. Testing process errors and their harms and consequences reported from family medicine practices: a study of the American Academy of Family Physicians National Research Network. Quality & Safety in Health Care. 2008;17:194-200. doi:10.1136/qshc.2006.021915.

Scientists shed light on festive medical myths (page 22)

Vreeman RC, Carroll AE. Seasonal medical myths that lack convincing evidence. BMJ. 2008 Dec 20-27;337:1442-3. doi:10.1136/bmj.39420 .420370.25.

Hospitalists—a new kind of doctor (page 24)

Hamel MB, Drazen JM, Epstein AM. The growth of hospitalists and the changing face of primary care. New England Journal of Medicine. 2009;360:1141-43.

Kuo Y-F, Sharma G, Freeman JL, Goodwin JS. Growth in the care of older patients by hospitalists in the United States. New England Journal of Medicine. 2009;360:1102-12.

Should we screen for childhood dyslipidemia? (page 29)

De Jongh S, Lilien MR, op't Roodt J, Stroes ES, Bakker HD, Kastelein JJ. Early statin therapy restores endothelial function in children with familial hypercholesterolemia. Journal of the American College of Cardiology. 2002;40:2117-21.

Friedman LA, Morrison JA, Daniels SR, McCarthy WF, Sprecher DL. Sensitivity and specificity of pediatric lipid determinations for adult lipid status: findings from the Princeton lipid research clinics prevalence program follow-up study. Pediatrics. 2006;118:165-72.

Haney EM, Huffman LH, Bougatsos C, Freeman M, Steiner RD, Nelson HD. Screening and treatment for lipid disorders in children and adolescents: systematic evidence review for the US Preventive Services Task Force. Pediatrics. 2007;120;e189-214.

Hickman TB, Briefel RR, Carroll MD, Rifkind BM, Cleeman JI, Maurer KR, et al. Distributions and trends of serum lipid levels among United States children and adolescents ages 4–19 years: data from the Third National Health and Nutrition Examination Survey. Preventive Medicine.1998;27:879-90.

Labarthe DR, Dai S, Fulton J. Cholesterol screening in children: insights from Project HeartBeat! and NHANES III. Progress in Pediatric Cardiology. 2003;17:169-78.

Lauer RM, Clarke WR. Use of cholesterol measurements in childhood for the prediction of adult hypercholesterolemia: the Muscatine study. JAMA. 1990;264:3034-8.

Stein EA, Illingworth DR, Kwiterovich PO Jr, Liacouras CA, Siimes MA, Jacobson MS, et al. Efficacy and safety of lovastatin in adolescent males with heterozygous familial hypercholesterolemia: a randomized controlled trial. JAMA. 1999;281:137-44.

Tanne JH. US pediatricians and cardiologists are criticized for recommending statins for children. BMJ. 2008;337:134. doi: 10.1136/ bmj.a813.

Webber LS, Srinivasan SR, Wattigney WA, Berenson GS. Tracking of serum and lipids and lipoproteins from childhood to adulthood: the Bogalusa heart study. American Journal of Epidemiology. 1991;133:884-99.

Wiegman A, Hutten BA, de Groot E, Rodenburg J, Bakker HD, Büller HR, et al. Efficacy and safety of statin therapy in children with familial hypercholesterolemia: a randomized controlled trial. JAMA. 2004;292:331-7.

Weighing prostate cancer screening recommendations (page 32)

Lin K, Lipsitz R, Miller T, Janakiraman S. Benefits and harms of prostate-specific antigen screening for prostate cancer: an evidence update for the US Preventive Services Task Force. Annals of Internal Medicine. 2008;149:192-9.

US Preventive Services Task Force. Screening for prostate cancer: US Preventive Services Task Force recommendation statement. Annals of Internal Medicine. 2008;149:185-91.

Shouting about shots (page 34)

Centers for Disease Control and Prevention. Measles—United States, January-July 2008. Morbidity and Mortality Weekly Report. 2008 Aug 22;57(33):893-6.

Mooney H. Government to offer MMR vaccine to all children in England. BMJ. 2008 Aug 11;337:370. doi: 10.1136/bmj.a1254.

The good news about the flu (page 37)

Centers for Disease Control and Prevention. The 2009 H1N1 pandemic: summary highlights, April 2009-April 2010 [Internet]. Atlanta: CDC [cited 2011 April 15]. Available from http://www.cdc.gov/h1n1flu /cdcresponse.htm

Does preventive care save money? (page 39)

Greenberg Quinlan Rosner Research. Americans overwhelmingly support investment in prevention [Internet]. Washington: Greenberg Quinlan Rosner Research and Public Opinion Strategies [cited 2011 April 15]. Available from: http://healthyamericans.org/assets/files/health-reform-poll-memo.pdf

Woolf SH. A closer look at the economic argument for disease prevention. JAMA. 2009;301(5):536-8. doi: 10.1001/jama.200951.

Debate over the H1N1 vaccine? There shouldn't be one (page 41)

Centers for Disease Control and Prevention. The 2009 H1N1 pandemic: summary highlights, April 2009-April 2010 [Internet]. Atlanta: CDC [cited 2011 April 15]. Available from: http://www.cdc.gov/h1n1flu/cdcresponse.htm

Mammograms, poor communication, and politics (page 43)

Nelson HD, Tyne K, Naik A, Bougatsos C, Chan BK, Humphrey, L. Screening for breast cancer: an update for the US Preventive Services Task Force. Annals of Internal Medicine. 2009;151:727-37.

Stein R. Breast exam guidelines now call for less testing. Washington Post [Internet]. 2009 Nov 17 [cited 2011 Jul 20]. Available from: http://www.washingtonpost.com/wp-dyn/content/article/2009/11/16/AR2009111602822.html

Steinhauer J. New mammogram advice finds a skeptical audience. New York Times [Internet]. 2009 Nov 17 [cited 2011 Jul 20]. Available from: http://www.nytimes.com/2009/11/18/health/18mammogram.html

US Preventive Services Task Force. Screening for breast cancer: US Preventive Services Task Force Recommendation Statement. Annals of Internal Medicine. 2009;151:716-26.

Is hypertension really a neglected disease? (page 46)

Committee on Public Health Priorities to Reduce and Control Hypertension in the US Population. A population-based policy and systems change approach to prevent and control hypertension. Washington: National Academies Press; 2010.

Roehr B. US doctors are lax in treating hypertension, report says. BMJ. 2010 Feb 22;340:444. doi: 10.113/bmj.c1074.

Depressed about depression (page 49)

American Psychiatric Association. APA releases new guidelines on the treatment of major depressive disorder [news release]. 2010 Oct 1 [cited 2011 Jul 20]. Available from: www.psych.org/MainMenu/Newsroom/NewsReleases/2010-News-Releases/New-MDD-Guidelines.aspx?FT=.pdf

Berwick DM. Screening in health fairs. A critical review of benefits, risks, and costs. JAMA 1985;254:1492-8.

Centers for Disease Control and Prevention. Current depression among adults—United States, 2006 and 2008. Morbidity and Mortality Weekly Report. 2010;59:1229-35.

Murray CJ, Lopez AD. Alternative projections of mortality and disability by cause 1990-2020: global burden of disease study. Lancet. 1997;349:1498-504.

National Depression Screening Day [Internet]. Wellesley (MA): Screening for Mental Health, Inc. [cited 2011 Apr 15]. Available from: www.mentalhealthscreening.org/programs/community/ndsd.aspx

O'Connor EA, Whitlock EP, Beil TL, Gaynes BN. Screening for depression in adult patients in primary care settings: a systematic evidence review. Annals of Internal Medicine. 2009:151:793-803.

US Preventive Services Task Force. Screening for depression. In: US Preventive Services Task Force. Guide to clinical preventive services. Baltimore (MD): Williams & Wilkins; 1989. p. 261-4.

US Preventive Services Task Force. Screening for depression in adults: US Preventive Force recommendation statement. Annals of Internal Medicine. 2009;151:784-92.

Screening for early detection of lung cancer (page 52)

Harris G. CT scans cut lung cancer deaths, study finds. New York Times. 2010 Nov 4;Sect. A:1 (col. 6).

National Cancer Institute. Lung cancer trial results show mortality benefit with low-dose CT [press release]. Bethesda (MD): National Cancer Institute [posted 2010 Nov 4; cited 2011 April 15]. Available from: http://www.cancer.gov/newscenter/pressreleases/2010/NLSTresultsRelease

AIDS at 30: A chance to treat is a chance to prevent (page 55)

Brown D. Tough decisions about money and treatment are ahead as AIDS turns 30. The Washington Post. 2011 May 31;Sect. D:1.

Fauci, AS. 30 years of AIDS. The Washington Post. 2011 May 29;Sect. A:17.

National Institutes of Health. Treating HIV-infected people with antiretrovirals significantly reduces transmission to partners [press release]. Bethesda (MD): National Institutes of Health. 2011 May 12 [cited 2011 June 15]. Available from: http://www.nih.gov/news/health/may2011/niaid-12.htm

Pneumocystis pneumonia—Los Angeles. Morbidity and Mortality Weekly Report. 1981;30(21):1-3.

Today's doctors' dilemma (page 61)

Agency for Healthcare Research and Quality. 2006 National Healthcare Quality Report. Rockville (MD): US Department of Health and Human Services, Agency for Healthcare Research and Quality; 2006 December. Publication No. AHRQ 07-0013.

Cutler D, Lleras-Muney A. Education and health: evaluating theories and evidence [Internet]. Cambridge [MA]: National Bureau of Economic Research; June 2006 [cited April 15, 2011]. Available from: http://www.chrp.org/pdf/Cutler_Lieras-Muney_Education_and_Health.pdf

Health I. In defense of a national sickness service. BMJ. 2007 Jan 4;334:19. doi: 10.1136/bmj.39080.481551.47.

Kolata G. A surprising secret to a long life: stay in school. New York Times [Internet]. 2007 Jan 3 [cited 2011 Jul 20]. Available from: http://www.nytimes.com/2007/01/03/health/03aging.html

Lleras-Muney A, Cutler D, Deaton A. The determinants of mortality. Journal of Economic Perspectives. 2006 summer;20(3):97-120.

McGinnis JM, Foege WH. Actual causes of death in the United States. JAMA. 1993;270(18):2207-12.

Shaw GB. The doctor's dilemma [Internet]. 1906. [Project Gutenberg Ebook cited 2009 March 26]. Available from: http://www.gutenberg.org/files/5070/5070-h/5070-h.htm

Woolf SH, Johnson RE. The break-even point: when medical advances are less important than improving the fidelity with which they are delivered. Annals of Family Medicine. 2005;3:545-552. doi: 10.1370/afm.406.

The cancer diagnosis that has gripped America (page 64)

Broder JM, Nagourney A. Heading toward 2008, Edwards says wife's cancer has returned. New York Times [Internet]. 2007 March 23; [cited 2011 Jul 20]. Available from: http://query.nytimes.com/gst/fullpage.html?res=9904 E7DC1530F930A15750C0A9619C8B63&ref=elizabethedwards

Grady D. "I don't expect my life to be significantly different," she says. New York Times [Internet]. 2007 March 23 [cited 2011 Jul 20]. Available from: http://www.nytimes.com/2007/03/23/us/politics/23illness.html?_ r=1&ref=elizabethedwards

Conflicts in office (page 67)

Tanne, JH. Former US surgeon general reveals extent of political pressure he was under. BMJ. 2007 July 19;335:114. doi: 10.1136/bmj.39279.393345. BE.

Lee, C. Ex-Surgeon general says White House hushed him. Washington Post. 2007 July 11;Sect. A:1.

What the candidates fail to mention (page 70)

Phillips RL, Starfield B. Why does a US primary care physician workforce crisis matter? American Family Physician. 2003 Oct 15;68(8):1494-500.

A cautionary tale for the presidential candidates (page 73)

Blackburn E. Bioethics and the political distortion of biomedical science. New England Journal of Medicine. 2004;350:1379-80.

Bloche MG. Health care disparities—science, politics, and race. New England Journal of Medicine. 2004;350:1568-70.

Bruni F, Lacey M. Bush acts to halt overseas spending tied to abortion. New York Times [Internet]. 2001 Jan 23 [cited 2011 Jul 20]. Available from: www.nytimes.com/2001/01/23/politics/23BUSH.html?ex=1224043200&e n=d4f89e6357e80d60&ei=5070

Davidoff F, Trussell J. Plan B and the politics of doubt. JAMA. 2006;296: 1775-8.

Rosenstock L. Protecting special interests in the name of "good science."
JAMA 2006;295:2407-10.

Steinbrook R. Science, politics, and federal advisory committees. New
England Journal of Medicine. 2004;350:1454-60.

Tanne, JH. Former US surgeon general reveals extent of political pressure he
was under. BMJ. 2007 July 19;335:114. doi: 10.1136/bmj.39279.393345.BE.

Union of Concerned Scientists. A to Z guide to political interference in
science [Internet]. Union of Concerned Scientists. [cited 2011 April 15].
Available from: http://www.ucsusa.org/scientific_integrity/abuses_of_
science/a-to-z-guide-to-political.html

What should the Surgeon General do? (page 76)

Profiles in science. The reports of the surgeon general. The 1964 report on
smoking and health. Bethesda (MD): US National Library of Medicine;
[cited 2011 Apr 15]. Available from. http://profiles.nlm.nih.gov
/ps/retrieve/Narrative/NN/p-nid/60

Zeleny J. CNN medical correspondent as surgeon general? 2009 Jan 6
[cited 2011 Apr 15]. In: New York Times. The caucus: the politics and
government blog of the Times. New York: New York Times Co.. Available
from: http://thecaucus.blogs.nytimes.com/2009/01/06/cnn-medical-
correspondent-as-surgeon-general/

The taxing case of Tom Daschle (page 79)

Daschle T, Lembrew JM, Greenberger SS. Critical: what we can do about the
health-care crisis. New York: Thomas Dunne, 2008.

Zeleny J. Tom Daschle withdraws as health nominee. 2009 Feb 3 [cited 2011
Apr 15]. In: New York Times. The caucus: the politics and government
blog of the Times. New York: New York Times Co. Available from:
http://thecaucus.blogs.nytimes.com/2009/02/03/tom-daschle-withdraws-
as-health-nominee/?scp=28&sq=daschle&st=nyt

The papal position on condoms and HIV (page 82)

Associated Press. Pope, in Africa, says condoms aren't the way to fight HIV.
New York Times [Internet]. 2009 Mar 17 [cited 2011 Jul 20]. Available
from: http://www.nytimes.com/2009/03/18/world/africa/18pope.html

Roehr B. Pope's claims that condoms exacerbate HIV and AIDS problem attract wide condemnation. BMJ. 2009;338:737. doi: 10.1136/bmj.b1206.

Russell S. Uganda's HIV rate drops, but not from abstinence. San Francisco Chronicle [Internet]. 2005 Feb 24 [cited 2011 Jul 20]. Available from: http://www.sfgate.com/cgi-bin/article.cgi?file=/c/a/2005/02/24/MNG2PBG3VF1.DTL

Weller SC, Davis-Beaty K. Condom effectiveness in reducing heterosexual HIV transmission. Cochrane Database of Systematic Reviews [Internet]. 2002 [cited 2011 Jul 20]. Issue 1. Art. No.: CD003255. doi: 10.1002/14651858.CD003255. Available from: http://www.mrw.interscience.wiley.com/cochrane/clsysrev/articles/CD003255/frame.html

The case of the sugar-sweetened beverage tax (page 85)

Brownell KD, Farley T, Willett WC, Popkin BM, Chaloupka FJ, Thompson JW, et al. The public health and economic benefits of taxing sugar-sweetened beverages. New England Journal of Medicine. 2009;361:1599-1605.

Craig T. Council all but kills soda tax. 2010 May 10 [cited 2011 April 15]. In: Washington Post. DC wire, news and notes on district politics [Internet]. Washington: Washington Post, c2010. Available from: http://voices.washingtonpost.com/dc/2010/05/council_all_but_kills_soda_tax.html

Hartocollis A. Failure of state soda tax plan reflects power of an anti-tax message. New York Times [Internet]. 2010 July 2 [cited 2011 Jul 20]. Available from: www.nytimes.com/2010/07/03/nyregion/03sodatax.html

Smoking or obesity: must we target only one? (page 88)

McGinnis JM, Foege WH. Actual causes of death in the United States. JAMA. 1993;270:2207-12.

Mokdad AH, Marks JS, Stroup DF, Gerberding JL. Actual causes of death in the United States, 2000. JAMA. 2004;291:1238-45.

Schroeder SA, Warner, KE. Don't forget tobacco. New England Journal of Medicine. 2010;363:201-4.

Sherry B, Blanck HM, Galuska DA, Pan L, Dietz WH, Balluz L. Vital signs: state-specific obesity prevalence among adults—United States, 2009. Morbidity and Mortality Weekly Report. 2010;59(3 Aug):1-3. Available from: www.cdc.gov/mmwr/preview/mmwrhtml/mm59e0803a1.htm

Tanne, JH. Michelle Obama launches programme to combat US childhood obesity. BMJ. 2010 (Feb 15);340:387. doi: 10.1136/bmj.c948.

Wilson D. A shift towards fighting fat. New York Times. 2010 Jul 28;Sect. B:1.

Guns don't kill crowds, people with semiautomatics do (page 91)

Collins B. A right to bear Glocks? New York Times [Internet]. 2011 Jan 9; [cited 2011 Jul 20]. Available from: http://www.nytimes.com/2011/01/10/opinion/10collins.html

Johnson K, Kovaleski SF, Frosch D, Lipton E. Suspect's odd behavior caused growing alarm. New York Times [Internet]. 2011 Jan 7 [cited 2011 Jul 20]. Available from: http://www.nytimes.com/2011/01/10/us/10shooter.html

Lipton E, Savage C, Shane S. Arizona suspect's recent acts offer hints of alienation. New York Times [Internet]. 2011 Jan 8 [cited 2011 Jul 20]. Available from: http://www.nytimes.com/2011/01/09/us/politics/09shooter.html

The rise and likely fall of Don Berwick (page 94)

Committee on Quality of Health Care in America, Institute of Medicine. Crossing the quality chasm: a new health system for the 21st century. Washington: National Academy Press; 2001.

Committee on Quality of Health Care in America, Institute of Medicine. To err is human: building a safer health system. Washington: National Academy Press; 1999.

Coughlin B. Sources: Dems giving up on Berwick. 2011 Mar 4 [cited 2011 April 15]. Politico.com [Internet]. Arlington (VA): Politico. Available from: http://www.politico.com/news/stories/0311/50698.html

Ignatius D. With Donald Berwick's appointment, the doctor is (finally) in. Washington Post. 2010 Jul 7; Sect. A:17.

Klein E. How much did Don Berwick get done? 2011 March 8 [cited 2011 Jun 21]. In: Washington Post. The Wonkbook [Internet]. Washington: Washington Post. Available from: http://voices.washingtonpost.com/ezra-klein/2011/03/how_much_did_don_berwick_get_d.html

Pear R. Rising calls to replace top man at Medicare. New York Times [Internet]. 2011 Mar 7 [cited 2011 Jul 20]. Available from: http://www.nytimes.com/2011/03/08/health/policy/08medicare.html

Our perfectly designed health care system (page 99)

Bodenheimer T. Primary care–will it survive? Annals of Internal Medicine. 2007;146:301-6.

Phillips RL. Primary care in the United States: problems and possibilities. BMJ. 2006;332:151.

Phillips RL, Starfield B. Why does a US primary care physician workforce crisis matter? American Family Physician. 2003 Oct 15;68(8):1494-1500.

Starr P. The social transformation of American medicine: the rise of a sovereign profession and the making of a vast industry. New York: Basic Books; 1984.

How to waste a billion dollars (page 102)

Avorn J. Debate about funding comparative-effectiveness research. New England Journal of Medicine. 2009 (May 7);360:1927-9.

Garber AM, Tunis SR. Does comparative-effectiveness research threaten personalized medicine? New England Journal of Medicine. 2009 (May 7);360:1925-7.

Naik AD, Petersen LA. The neglected purpose of comparative-effectiveness research. New England Journal of Medicine. 2009 (May 7);360:1929-31.

Partnership to improve patient care [Internet]. Washington: The Partnership [cited 2011 April 15]. Available from: http://www.improvepatientcare.org

The gatekeeper and the wizard, redux (page 108)

Herd B, Herd A, Mathers N. The wizard and the gatekeeper: of castles and contracts. BMJ. 1995;310:1042-4.

Mathers N, Hodgkin P. The gatekeeper and the wizard: a fairy tale. BMJ. 1989;298:172-4

Mathers N, Usherwood T. The gatekeeper and the wizard revisited. BMJ. 1992;304:969-71.

Phillips RL. Primary care in the United States: problems and possibilities. BMJ. 2006;332:151.

Phillips RL, Starfield B. Why does a US primary care physician workforce crisis matter? Am Fam Physician. 2003 Oct 15;68(8):1494-1500.

All or nothing at all? (page 110)

Side-by-side comparison of major health care reform proposals [Internet]. Washington: Kaiser Family Foundation; 2009 [cited 2001 Apr 15]. Available from: http://www.kff.org/healthreform/upload/healthreform_sbs_full.pdf

US health care reform is in the waste can (page 113)

Pear R, Herszenhorn DM. A new search for consensus on health care bill New York Times [Internet]. 2010 Jan 21 [cited 2011 Jul 20]. Available from: http://www.nytimes.com/2010/01/22/health/policy/22health.html

Stolberg SG, Herszenhorn DM. Obama weighs paring goals for health bill. New York Times [Internet]. 2010 January 20 [cited 2011 Jul 20]. Available from: http://www.nytimes.com/2010/01/21/health/policy/21health.html

Prevention and the new health reform act (page 116)

Alderman L. For many, health law offers a chance for preventive care. New York Times. 2010 Apr 10;Sect. B:6 (col.1).

Health reform resource center. What's in the Affordable Care Act? [Internet]. New York: The Commonwealth Fund [cited 2011 Apr 15]. Available from: http://www.commonwealthfund.org/Health-Reform/Health-Reform-Resource.aspx

Himmelstein DU, Woolhandler S. Obama's reform: no cure for what ails us. BMJ. 2010 March 30;340:742. doi: 10.1136/bmj.c1778.

PCORI—odd name, important job, potential trouble (page 119)

Elshaug AG, Garber AM. How CER could pay for itself—insights from vertebral fracture treatments. New England Journal of Medicine. 2011;364:1390-3.

Institute of Medicine. Initial national priorities for comparative effectiveness research. Washington: National Academies Press; 2009.

Kamerow, DB. How to waste a billion dollars. BMJ. 2009(June 20);338:1473.

The Patient Protection and Affordable Care Act, Pub. L. No. 111-148 (March 23, 2010).

Partnership to Improve Patient Care [Internet]. Washington: The Partnership [cited 2011 April 15]. Available from: http://www.improvepatientcare.org

Wall Street Journal (editorial). The pro-diabetes board. 2011 Mar 18. Available from: http://online.wsj.com/article/SB10001424052748704662604576202883913468422.html

Killing me softly (page 125)

Weil E. The needle and the damage done. New York Times Magazine. 2007 Feb 11 [cited 2011 Jul 20]. Available from: http://www.nytimes.com/2007/02/11/magazine/11injection.t.html

Gawande A. When law and ethics collide—why physicians participate in executions. New England Journal of Medicine. 2006 (Mar 23);354:1221-9.

The Medicare Part D signup blues (page 128)

Medicare plan finder. Baltimore (MD): Centers for Medicare & Medicaid Services. [cited 2011 April 15]. Available from: https://www.medicare.gov/find-a-plan/questions/home.aspx

Who wrote that article? (page 130)

DeAngelis CD, Fontanarosa PB. Impugning the integrity of medical science—the adverse effects of industry influence. JAMA. 2008:288(15):1833-5.

Ross JS, Hill KP, Egilman DS, Krumholz HM. Guest authorship and ghostwriting in publications related to rofecoxib. JAMA. 2008;299(15):1800-12.

Smith R. The trouble with medical journals. New York: Oxford University Press; 2006.

Aesculapius on a plane (page 133)

Dowdall N. Is there a doctor on the aircraft? Top 10 in-flight medical emergencies. BMJ. 2000;321:1336-7.

Gendreau MA, DeJohn C. Responding to medical events during commercial airline flights. New England Journal of Medicine. 2002;346:1067-73.

Qureshi A, Porter KM. Emergencies in the air. Emerg Med J. 2005;22:658-9.

Placebo pills for children (page 136)

Aschwanden C. Experts question placebo pills for children. New York Times [Internet]. 2008 May 27 [cited 2011 Jul 21]. Available from: http://www. nytimes.com/2008/05/27/health/27plac.html

Balint M. The doctor, his patient and the illness. London: Churchill Livingstone; 2000.

Kaptchuk TJ, Kelley JM, Conboy LA, Davis RB, Kerr CE, Jacobson EE, et al. Components of placebo effect: randomised controlled trial in patients with irritable bowel syndrome. BMJ. 2008(May 3);336: 999-1003. doi: 10.1136/bmj.39524.439618.25.

Obecalp—standardized pharmaceutical grade placebo [Internet]. Baltimore (MD): Efficacy Brands [cited 2011 April 11]. Available from: http://www. inventedbyamother.com

Pittroff R, Rubenstein I. The thinking doctor's guide to placebos. BMJ. 2008(May 3);336:1020. doi: 10.1136/bmj.39564.454502.C2.

No gifts, please, we're doctors (page 139)

Harris G. Institute of Medicine calls for doctors to stop taking gifts from drug makers. New York Times [Internet]. 2009 Apr 28 [cited 2011 Jul 21]. Available from: http://www.nytimes.com/2009/04/29/health/policy /29drug.html

Lo B, Field MJ, Editors; Committee on Conflict of Interest in Medical Research, Education, and Practice; Institute of Medicine. Conflict of interest in medical research, education, and practice. Washington: National Academies Press; 2009.

About the Author

Douglas Kamerow is a family physician and a specialist in preventive medicine. After graduating from Harvard College, the University of Rochester Medical School, and Johns Hopkins University School of Hygiene and Public Health, he spent 20 years in the Commissioned Corps of the US Public Health Service. In the PHS he worked as a general practitioner in the National Health Service Corps, as a researcher at the National Institute of Mental Health, and in health policy and leadership positions at both the Office of the Assistant Secretary for Health and at the Agency for Healthcare Research and Quality. He retired from the PHS in 2001 with the rank of Assistant Surgeon General.

Since then, Dr. Kamerow has been a chief scientist at the nonpartisan research institute RTI International, an editor of the international medical journal *BMJ*, and a professor at Georgetown University, where he teaches medical students and family medicine residents. Starting in 2007, he wrote the health and health care commentaries in this book, which appeared first in the *BMJ* or on National Public Radio (NPR).

Dr. Kamerow lives in Washington, DC, with his wife, Celia Shapiro, and their three almost-grown children.